JA HERBS

40 Jamaican Medicinal Herbs

Kukuwa Abba

D1641233

KUUMBA BOOKS

First published 2016 by Kuumba Books

ISBN number: 978 1 78645 075 3

Editing and typesetting by Beaten Track Publishing
Burscough. L40 7TW. United Kingdom
Website: www.beatentrackpublishing.com

NOTE: This book is for information only and is not intended to be a substitute for medical services. Neither the author nor the publisher is liable for any misuse of the information provided. Readers are advised to seek help from a qualified health practitioner if they experience any health problems.

Acknowledgements

All thanks and praises to HIM Haile Selassie 1 for the inspiration, the guidance and the fortitude to make this journey.

Give thanks to my children and grandchildren, for their love and support, to my partner for all his support and patience, to my parents and ancestors, without whom I would not be. Thanks to all my sistren and brethren for their support and encouragement over the years. Special thanks to Brother Napthali, for his invaluable help in bringing this book to life.

I owe a debt of gratitude to all the healers who have shared their knowledge and experience with me over the years, especially Nanny Ivy and others in the hills of Portland, who have shared with me the legacy of our herbal culture.

To all who participated in the journey, give thanks!

Kukuwa Abba

Contents

Introduction

Blessed love!

If you are reading this, it means that you have bought, borrowed, or otherwise got hold of a copy of JA Herbs. Give thanks.

JA Herbs represents a long and fruitful journey. Over 30 years ago, after years of living in the big cities of the North, I returned to Jamaica; to be precise, I returned to my maternal family roots in Portland. Against a backdrop of mindless political violence and a commitment to the teachings of Haile Selassie 1 and Marcus Garvey, I went with my family to live in the hills of Portland. We were miles from the nearest anything, and like babes in the woods, we learned about living in our new environment and coping with the reality of living off the land.

It was here that I developed an interest in the plant life of those blessed hills, and the first thing I needed to do was to be able to identify one green thing from another. Coming as I did from a cosmopolitan background, this was a real challenge. I am still indebted to Ras Micky Peters (now deceased) and Bro Teeko Thompson for those early and important lessons of life in the hills.

Having two young daughters and living miles from a doctor or hospital meant that I had to learn natural first aid when they had colds, hurt themselves or when we adults had our health problems. Somehow we survived, and after more than three years, we left the hills. I regard those three years as my PhD in survival and at least my first degree in herbs.

In the early '90s, I returned to Europe and eventually settled in London. I developed my interest in healing and expanded my knowledge of the various healing arts and sciences. I spent over ten years working in the National Health Service (NHS) in the preventative and public health sector, and it was this experience that convinced me that alternative or complementary therapies have a vital role to play in maintaining and improving people's health.

I used the opportunity while living in Europe to gather information on a variety of these therapies, and found that my real passion was for herbal healing. However, most of the information on herbal medicine related to European, North American, Chinese or Indian traditions of herbal healing.

On my return to Portland in 2004, I embarked on my mission to document information on herbal healing in Jamaica. To my surprise, I found that the knowledge about our own healing herbs was being lost with each passing decade.

Bush medicine, as we call it in Jamaica, was losing ground rapidly to Western pharmaceuticals. In our rush to be modern, we had discarded our original knowledge of self-help with herbs in favour of a trip to the pharmacy.

As I went about studying the local herbs, I realised how much there was to learn. Walking around in my community of Nonsuch and the neighbouring Look Out area of Portland, I realised that not only was the knowledge being lost but the very herbs themselves were becoming endangered. With the spread of modern farming techniques, local farmers were being encouraged to use more products ending in 'cide', which, as we know, means death. So they use herbicides that get rid of all 'weeds' as well as anything else that gets in the way of the spray, insecticides to get rid of 'pests' and fungicides to get rid of fungi on crops. The debate around organic farming points clearly to the fact that while these various '-cides' seem to increase crop yields in the short term, they cost the earth and possibly our health in the long run.

Most of the local farmers can be described as subsistence farmers, and they will, of course, opt for whatever is likely to increase their income and improve their lives. If the new methods bring in more money, then it is difficult to insist that they should return to what was their original ways of farming. Enlightened self-interest often works where the big-stick approach fails. If the farmers and others in the community knew the value of some of the weeds they were 'nuking' then maybe they might be persuaded to be more careful in their use of the 'cides'.

Let me state up front that I am not a botanist nor am I medically trained, but I have the necessary skills and experience to gather information on the herbs, appraise the information and present it in an accessible form. I also have experience of using many of these herbs both for self-help and to treat others. I have decided to focus on herbs that have proven healing properties, and I have only included herbs for which I have information about the plant chemicals they contain and any research undertaken on them.

All of these herbs are used in various herbal systems; sometimes they are used in the same way that we use them in Jamaica, but in many cases they are used for very different health problems. This has been a real journey of discovery for me as I have unearthed both local and international research on some of our lesser known herbs, vines, roots, seeds and barks. It just confirmed for me the need to conserve and preserve our natural heritage, if for no other reason than we might be destroying plants that could save us.

There is still a tremendous amount of work to be done in this regard, and I hope that our academic institutions will continue to undertake more research into the medicinal benefits of local herbs. A significant amount of work has already been done but there is scope for so much more. My long-term hope is that Jamaica will create a profitable and sustainable herbal industry, with the development of pharmaceutical, nutraceutical, cosmetic and other economically viable products from our herbal wealth.

I hope that enterprising companies or groups will find ways to turn research into economic opportunities for rural communities in particular and for the general population. I sincerely hope that this book can contribute in some way to the achievement of Jamaica's sustainable development goals.

The Format of JA Herbs

I have had many discussions with myself and significant others about how to present the information that I have gathered. In the end, I have tried to straddle a number of approaches in the format and that, I know, can carry its own challenges.

Firstly, for the purpose of this book, the word 'herb' is used to include leafy plants, roots of plants, vines, trees or seeds of plants or fruits.

Anyone who has tried to gather information on herbs, especially the lesser known ones, will know that the names of many herbs vary from place to place. The local or **Common Name** of the herb is given as the headline entry; again, it must be stated that there can be a number of local names for a given plant, and in some cases, the same name is used for different plants.

The **Botanical or Latin name** of the plant makes life a little easier, but there are cases in which botanists disagree on classifications and names. One of the main aims of the book was to make these plants easily recognisable by having a picture of each (in colour). This can assist identification of the herbs when descriptions and unclear illustrations are less than helpful. If nothing else, I hope that I have got this right.

Given practical constraints, I have had to balance how much information is included in JA Herbs. In relation to the particular herb the **Parts Used** are highlighted. I wanted to get a balance between information on **Traditional Uses** and **Modern Research and Uses**. It is important to recognise how herbs have been used over time in particular cultures; to acknowledge the wisdom of the ancestors. It is also important to realise that knowledge is increasing and that research into herbs can give us new insight into the way in which a particular herb works and to identify what the active **Plant Chemicals** are in the herb. The plant chemicals are given as compounds as it would be difficult to list all the chemicals in any plant. These are not listed in any particular order.

Where appropriate, there is a note of **Caution** on using a particular herb. With the increase of chronic, non-communicable diseases such as diabetes and high blood pressure, especially in Jamaica and internationally, it is important that we are aware that herbs can interact with pharmaceutical drugs that have been prescribed for such conditions. There is also information on other health conditions where it might be inadvisable to use particular herbs. The increased use of over-the-counter (OTC) medicines is also a factor, and it is useful to know when it might not be a good idea to use herbs alongside these OTC drugs.

I have included information on **Other Uses** that the various herbs have, as this highlights economic and other potential benefits. Hopefully, this will encourage the preservation of these plants for those who would otherwise have little interest in their medicinal value.

There is also a quick reference on the treatment of **Common Health Conditions** with the various herbs included in the book. This is intended to be a summary of both traditional and research-based uses; however, it is not intended to be a substitute for medical treatment or consultation with a health professional, and no claims are being made in that regard. In fact, the need to seek professional help is stressed throughout the book.

There are trained, qualified herbal healers and other health professionals who can provide services for people who have any health concerns. For many less serious and common ailments, herbs can be useful, if used safely and with the same caution and common sense you would apply to using over-the-counter drugs.

A quick overview of **How to Use Herbs** is also included, so that readers can be guided on the best way to prepare and use herbs. A **Glossary of Terms** used in herbal medicine has also been provided.

JA HERBS

Descriptions

Traditional Uses

Modern Research and Uses

Plant Chemicals

ANNATTO – Bixa orellana – Bixaceae

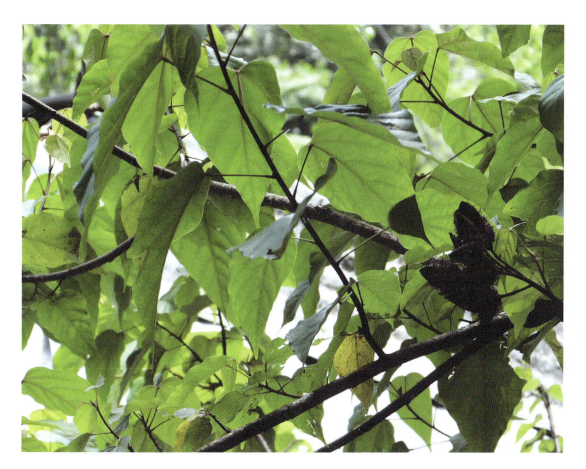

Other Names: Achiote; Bija; Roucou; Uruku; Lipstick Tree; Achuete

Brief Description

Annatto is a shrub or small tree that is native to South and Central America and the Caribbean. It was introduced into the Philippines by the Spanish and now grows in various parts of Indo-China. The tree can grow up to ten metres in height and bears hundreds of heart-shaped prickly pods, which contain many tiny red seeds.

Parts Used: Leaves; Roots; Seeds; Oil

Traditional Uses

Annatto is not known as a traditional healing herb in Jamaica; it was grown mainly for culinary use (see below). In other parts of the Caribbean, annatto is more widely used for a number of health conditions. The roots are infused in either water or rum for diabetes, skin problems and sexually transmitted infections. In Surinam, a leaf decoction is drunk to relieve nausea and vomiting.

Annatto is used as a herbal remedy in many countries in South and Central America, where the plant is indigenous. For example, in Mexico and Columbia, a paste made from the seeds is taken internally to treat liver disorders, cassava poisoning and snake bites. Annatto leaves are a popular traditional remedy in Peru for a wide range of conditions, including heartburn, liver and stomach problems, prostate disorders, skin infections and as a diuretic. The leaves and roots of the annatto plant are used in Brazil to lower fevers, to treat colic, vomiting, nausea and as a mild laxative. The seed paste is still used in parts of South America as a low-cost insect repellent, particularly against mosquitos.

In many parts of Southeast Asia, annatto leaves are used for fevers, to treat digestive problems, dysentery, cystitis and other inflammatory conditions. In the Philippines and Vietnam, a paste of the seeds and a leaf decoction are applied to burns to reduce scarring and blisters.

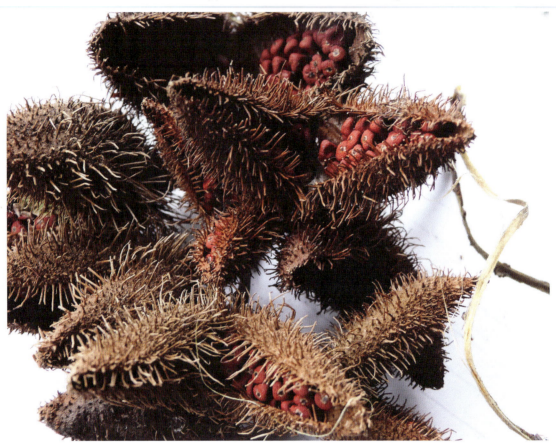

Modern Research and Uses

Recent studies have shown that extracts from the leaves of the annatto plant exhibited anti-inflammatory and anti-microbial activity. In one experiment, an annatto extract proved to be more effective than gentamicin sulphate against various microbes, while in another study, it had limited effects against gonorrhoea, E. coli and Staphylococcus aureus. In animal tests, a water-and-alcohol extract of annatto leaves demonstrated protective effects on stomach lining. A study carried out in Nigeria showed that regular consumption of annatto seed protected mice against a range of liver disorders. This was confirmed by research in Bangladesh using an ethanol extract of annatto leaves.

Research carried out at the University of the West Indies concluded that a crude extract of annatto leaves reduced blood sugar levels, and this result has been confirmed in a number of subsequent studies in animals. Annatto has also demonstrated significant diuretic activity that can contribute to lowering blood pressure and supports traditional use of the herb for increasing urination.

The oil from annatto seeds is reported to have very high levels of tocotrienols and extremely low or zero levels of tocopherols, when compared to other plant sources of these vitamin E compounds, such as soya, grain bran and palm oil. Latest research has shown that tocotrienols have significant antioxidant properties that are very effective in reducing cardiovascular risk factors, such as high cholesterol and lipid levels and can also inhibit the growth of tumours.

An ethanol extract of annatto leaves given to mice resulted in the mice having fewer symptoms of the effects of drug-induced cardiac disease. The extract also demonstrated strong cardio-protective effects when administered to mice even after they had developed cardiac disease.

The traditional use of annatto seed paste to repel insects has been validated by laboratory tests. The development of commercial repellents made from annatto could benefit large numbers of people who face health risks from exposure to mosquitos. Annatto grows in countries where the Aedes aegypti species that cause serious illnesses like dengue fever, yellow fever and the Chikungunya and Zika viruses are prevalent.

Plant Chemicals

Chemical compounds in annatto include: flavonoids; steroids; terpenoids; phenols; alkaloids; carotenoids; glycosides; tannins.

Other Uses

A paste made from the ground annatto seeds has been used traditionally in South America and the Caribbean as body paint and food colouring.

A pulp made from the seeds is used commercially for colouring in a wide range of industries. Annatto paste is used mainly in the food industry where it is added to a variety of foodstuffs needing yellow or orange colouring, such as margarine, cheese, oils, popcorn and smoked fish. In Europe, it is seen on food labels as E160b.

The oil is being increasingly used in the cosmetic industry due to its emollient and antioxidant properties. Annatto also adds a rich colour to cosmetic products ranging from soaps and creams to shampoos.

Annatto paste is used in the production of paints, lacquers and varnishes and as a natural dye for wool and other fabrics.

Caution!

Although annatto is effective in reducing blood sugar levels and to some extent blood pressure, mainly due to its strong diuretic action, people with diabetes and hypertension should use annatto internally under the supervision of a qualified health professional.

Recently, there have been growing concerns, particularly in Europe, about allergic reactions to annatto, which is widely used in the food industry. Some companies now use beta-carotene (E160a) instead of annatto as a natural food colourant.

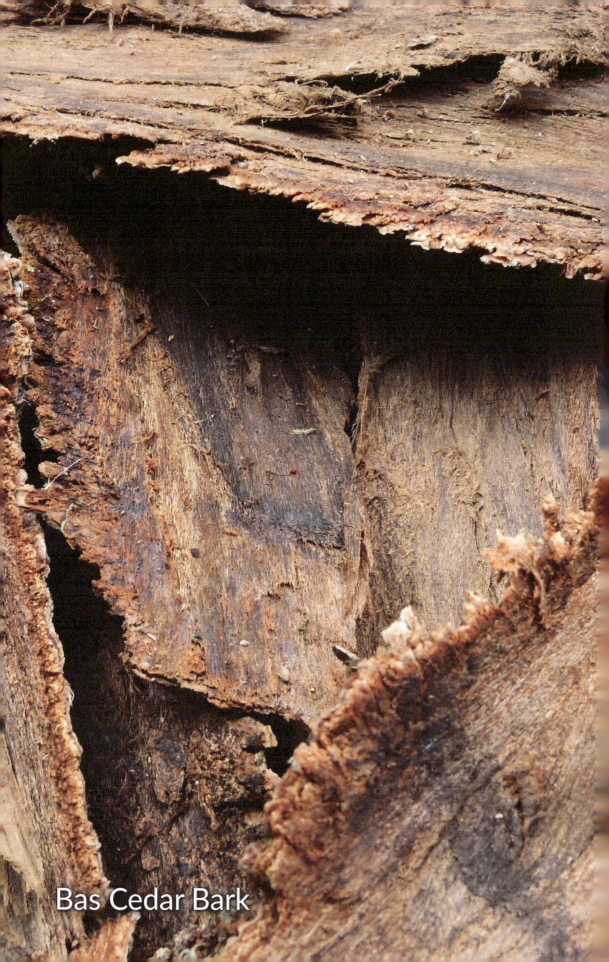

Bas Cedar Bark

BAS CEDAR – Guazuma ulmifolia – Sterculiaceae

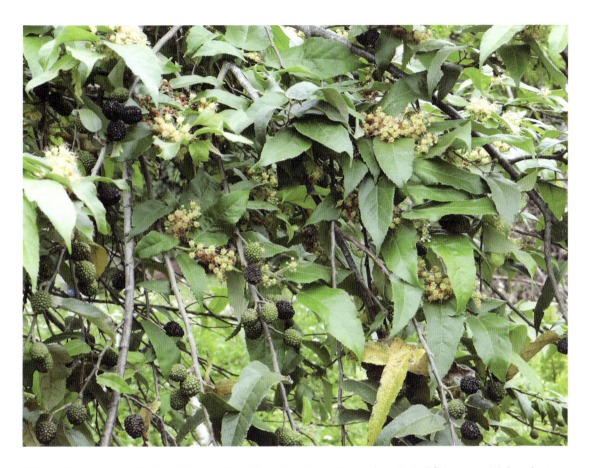

Other Names: Bay Cedar; West Indian Elm; Guazima; Mutamba; Bois D'Homme; Mahot-hetre; Pigeon Wood; Rudraksha; Honey Fruit Tree

Brief Description

Bas Cedar is native to the tropical regions of the Americas, but now grows in many tropical parts of the world. The tree can grow to a height of 20 metres or more, with leaves that are oblong or slightly oval. Bas cedar bears very pale yellowish flowers, which give way to small green fruits that have a very rough skin and turn dark brown when ripe. The bark of the tree has a rough, fissured texture.

Parts Used: Bark; Leaves; Roots; Fruits

Traditional Uses

In Jamaica, various parts of the bas cedar tree have been traditionally used both internally and externally. Scrapings of the inner bark are applied like a plaster to heal cuts and sores; a decoction of the bark is also used for the same purpose. Bas cedar bark is boiled as a remedy for chesty coughs, diarrhoea and urinary complaints. The fruits and their seeds can be boiled together with irish moss to make a thick porridge-like beverage, which is reputed to help men with sexual weakness. Bas cedar bark is still used as an ingredient in some roots tonics that are popular in Jamaica.

In other Caribbean countries, the crushed fruits are decocted and used to treat colds, diarrhoea, menstrual disorders and sexually transmitted infections. The leaves and young fruit shoots are also used for various complaints, including sore throats, fever and externally for skin problems.

Bas cedar is used in Central and South America for a wide range of conditions, such as diarrhoea, haemorrhaging, uterine pain and fibroids, childbirth, stomach inflammation, sexually transmitted infections, prostate problems and skin diseases. A decoction and syrup made from bas cedar is a popular remedy for coughs, colds and bronchitis. In Brazil, it is said to be effective for detoxifying the blood, for asthma, and for liver problems and has long been regarded there as an effective treatment for hair loss. In Indonesian traditional medicine, bas cedar is used for fevers, obesity, coughs, diarrhoea and abdominal pains.

Modern Research and Uses

Research on bas cedar has been ongoing for almost forty years, and in that time, many of the active plant chemicals found in both leaf and bark extracts have been confirmed as having antibacterial, antioxidant and antiviral properties. High levels of tannin in the bark are thought to be one of the reasons for bas cedar's anti-diarrhoeal effects.

Recent research has highlighted the broad benefits of one particular chemical, procyanidin B-2, which has shown promising signs of anti-tumour and anti-cancer activity. Procyanidins are also thought to be responsible for bas cedar's effectiveness in lowering blood pressure by widening blood vessels. Research has also confirmed that procyanidin B-2 can increase hair growth, which is one of the traditional uses for bas cedar.

Bas cedar has demonstrated effectiveness in reducing blood-sugar in lab tests, but further studies are needed. Bas cedar was also found to be beneficial in treating asthma and other upper respiratory disorders, confirming another traditional use of the plant. Recent studies have pointed to bas cedar being effective in weight loss, which could have significant benefits in improving overall health and wellbeing for overweight and obese people.

Plant Chemicals

The main chemical compounds in bas cedar include: steroids; alkaloids; saponins; tannins; phenols; glycosides; flavonoids; terpenoids.

Caution!

Do not use bas cedar when pregnant. People who have high blood pressure should use bas cedar under professional supervision.

BITTER ALBUT – *Neurolaena lobata* – Asteraceae

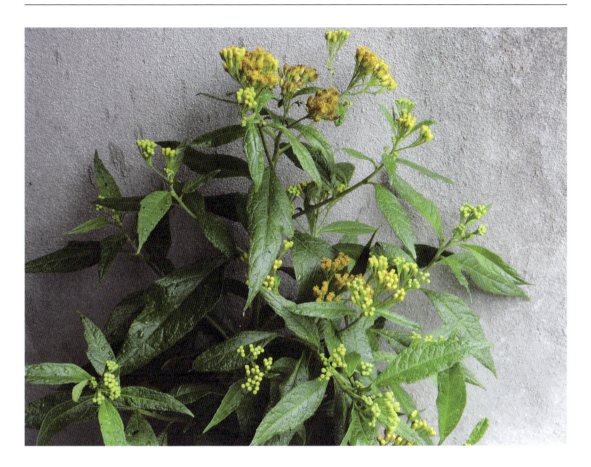

Other names: Golden Bitters; Jackass Bitters; Tres Puntas; Zeb a Pik; Alligator Foot; Kayabim; Cow Gall Bitters; Bushy Fleabane; Sour Bush; Wild Tobacco; Halbert Weed

Brief Description

Bitter albut is a common tropical plant growing by the wayside or in cleared forests. It can grow up to four metres in height and has spreading branches with distinctive three-pointed leaves and bears bright yellow flowers.

Parts Used: Leaves and Roots

Traditional Uses

Bitter albut is used in Jamaica to cleanse and purify the blood and is regarded as particularly effective because of its very bitter taste. It is also used for stomach problems, including diarrhoea; for colds, fevers and externally on sores that are hard to heal. In other Caribbean islands, bitter albut is used in similar ways and also for ringworm and chronic chest coughs.

In Central and South America, it is known as 'tres puntas' and is regarded as a cure-all. Bitter albut is mainly used in those countries to treat malaria, diabetes, biliousness, stomach pains and amoebic dysentery. It is also said to be effective for uterine congestion and to cleanse internal organs. In Guatemala, bitter albut leaves are rubbed and the juice applied directly onto the skin to treat fungal and other skin infections and ingested for removing intestinal parasites. The leaves are traditionally decocted or soaked in wine or alcohol and water and taken as required. A leaf decoction can be used to wash hair in cases of lice infestation.

Modern Research and Uses

Recent research has confirmed many of the traditional uses of bitter albut. The active plant chemicals are reported to be effective in treating malaria and fevers. Bitter albut has also been proven to be a blood purifier, an anti-fungal, and is particularly useful for intestinal worms and dysentery.

Hypoglycaemic activity in bitter albut has been researched with encouraging results, and studies have also reported bitter albut's effectiveness as an anti-protozoal. In laboratory tests in Mexico, bitter albut inhibited the growth of the protozoa: Leishmania mexicana, Trichomanas vaginalis and Trypanosoma cruzi, which cause Chagas disease.

In another study in mice, an alcohol-and-water extract from bitter albut leaves reduced swelling and demonstrated significant analgesic properties. Bitter albut also compared favourably with acetaminophen in reducing fever in mice, confirming one of the main traditional uses of the herb. A recent laboratory study found that a methylene chloride extract of bitter albut inhibited the growth of malignant cancer cells of both human and mouse origin. The plant's anti-inflammatory properties have been confirmed, which, combined with its analgesic effects, indicate that bitter albut could be useful in treating such conditions as arthritis and other joint problems.

Plant Chemicals

Plant chemicals in bitter albut include: coumarins; flavonoids; alkaloids; terpenoids; tannins; saponins.

Other Uses

Traditionally, bitter albut has been applied to the skin as an insect repellent. A decoction of the whole plant is also used to minimise insect and parasite infestation in animals and can also be applied to plants.

CARRY MI SEED – Phyllanthus niruri – Euphorbiaceae

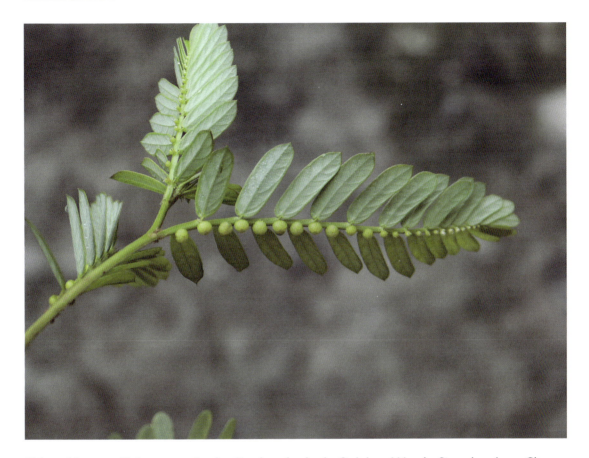

Other Names: Pickney-pon-back; Seed-under-leaf; Quinine Weed; Stonebreaker; Chanca Piedra; Arranca-pedras; Punarnava; Grain en bas; Quinine Creole; Ombatoatshi; Hurricane Weed; Sampa-sampalukan

Brief Description

Carry mi seed is a small erect herb, which is native to tropical parts of the world from the Amazon and Caribbean to India and China. It grows wild as a weed and is noticeable by the seeds which grow on the underside of the compound leaves. The male plant is greener in appearance than the female which has a reddish tinge in the stems. The female plant is said to be medicinally more potent than the male.

Parts Used: Roots; Leaves; Whole plant

Traditional Uses

Carry mi seed is rarely used today as a healing herb in Jamaica, but in the past was mainly used for fevers, diabetes, genito-urinary infections, dysentery, jaundice, and boiled with milk weed to treat gonorrhoea. In the Eastern Caribbean, carry mi seed is used traditionally for fevers and diarrhoea.

Carry mi seed has a long history in herbal medicine systems worldwide and is used for a variety of complaints in India and China. Carry mi seed is used in those healing systems to treat liver disorders, including jaundice, urinary infections and viral illnesses, such as colds and flu. It is also applied to sores and snake bites. In India, carry mi seed is reputed to be effective in treating inflammatory disorders such as prostatitis and cystitis.

In South and Central America the herb is known as 'chanca piedra' or 'stonebreaker', due to its reputation for treating kidney stones. A decoction of the roots is reportedly effective for jaundice and biliousness, similar to the herb's traditional use in Eastern medicine.

Modern Research and Uses

Recent research has confirmed the traditional use of the plant for liver and urinary disorders. Carry mi seed can protect the liver and is useful in treating viral Hepatitis B. There is strong evidence of the plant's effectiveness in treating kidney stones; there is, however, less evidence of its effect on gall-bladder stones.

One study of Ghanaian plants found that carry mi seed had significant antibacterial activity against Staphylococcus aureus, including the multi-resistant strain, commonly referred to as MRSA, and also demonstrated strong anti-candida activity. In another study, an extract of carry mi seed inhibited the growth of three types of bacteria which affect the stomach.

In tests on mice, carry mi seed had significant diuretic activity comparable to hydrochlorothiazide, a commonly prescribed diuretic. The herb has also shown promising results in stimulating the immune system, reducing tumours and limiting fertility. Carry mi seed has anti-inflammatory properties, which might explain its effectiveness in conditions such as cystitis, prostatitis, urinary tract infections (UTIs) and sexually transmitted infections (STIs).

Traditional use of carry mi seed for colds and flu has been confirmed by recent research on the plant's antiviral properties. Geranin, one of the chemicals in the plant, is said to be seven times more potent as a pain reliever than aspirin and acetaminophen. The properties of some of the plant chemicals that have been identified, might explain carry mi seed's effectiveness in reducing fevers, including its traditional use in treating malaria.

In laboratory experiments, an alkaloidal extract of carry mi seed was reported to have inhibitory effects on HIV in human cell lines. Further research is required to identify and isolate the active chemicals in the herb which could prove useful in the development of prevention and treatment options for HIV and AIDS.

Plant Chemicals

The plant chemicals in carry mi seed include: saponins; flavonoids; terpenoids; lignans; coumarins; phenols; tannins; glucosides; alkaloids.

Other Uses

A strong decoction of the leaves and stems is used in India to dye cotton fabric black.

Caution!

This plant offers a number of benefits for people suffering from a variety of diseases. However, it is important to take care when using carry mi seed, as it can interact with other medication. People with diabetes, high blood pressure and heart problems should have their condition monitored by a health professional if using this herb. Carry mi seed should not to be used in pregnancy!

CERASSEE – *Momordica charantia* – Cucurbitaceae

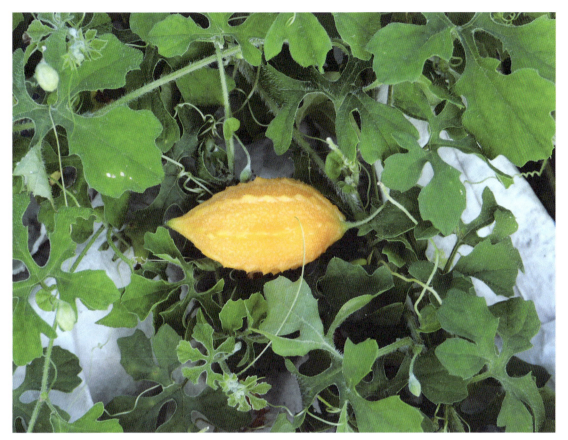

Other Names: Bitter Melon; Maiden Apple; Paoka; Pomme Coolee; Karela; Salsamino; Pava-aki; Bitter Gourd; Ampalaya; Ku Gua; Cocouli; Sorossie

Brief Description

Cerassee is a creeping vine, which is native to Asia but now grows in many tropical countries. The plant has lobed leaves and bears pale yellow flowers and a green fruit that turns orange when ripe, with the seeds covered in red pulp.

Parts used: Seeds; Leaves; Vines; Fruits

Traditional Uses

In Jamaica, cerassee is used mainly for colds, fevers, stomach problems and to cleanse and detoxify the body. It is particularly valued for purges and treating skin problems. Cerassee is also used to treat diabetes. In the past, people were advised not to use it for this purpose, as it could mask true sugar levels in blood and urine. Cerassee is also thought to be effective in treating liver problems, especially jaundice.

In the Eastern Caribbean, cerassee is reputed to be effective in treating menstrual problems, skin problems, such as rashes and acne (used internally and externally), and as a purgative.

In the Philippines, dried powdered leaf or a decoction of the root is applied externally for haemorrhoids, and juice from the green fruit is used for chronic inflammation of the colon and for dysentery.

Cerassee is used in Central and South America for many of the same conditions as above, but is also popularly used to treat malaria, measles, eczema and as an aid in childbirth.

Modern Research and Uses

Most of the research on cerassee has focused on its ability to reduce blood sugar. There have only been a few human trials examining the effects of cerassee on diabetes, but these have been inconclusive. Results have shown that the green fruits are more effective in reducing blood sugar than the rest of the plant. Hopefully, further studies will provide more evidence on this issue. In an experiment with diabetic rats, cerassee was reported to be effective in reducing cholesterol levels in the animals.

There has also been research into the potential of certain plant chemicals in cerassee on human immunodeficiency virus (HIV). Cerassee contains proteins, called momorcharins, which in laboratory tests were effective in blocking both the infection of cells by HIV and inhibiting replication of the virus. Other research in vitro has reported cerassee's effectiveness against various cancers including leukaemia. The theory is that plant chemicals in cerassee can promote immune function and increase resistance to viral and bacterial infections.

Cerassee can be effective in treating stomach problems, including those caused by bacterial infections, and could also be useful for colitis and other inflammation of the gut. Some of the same properties in cerassee that are effective on internal conditions are also useful for skin conditions, such as psoriasis, acne, haemorrhoids, and ringworm. Some studies and anecdotal evidence suggest that extracts from the roots and fruits of the cerassee can cause abortions and can affect fertility in both men and women.

Plant Chemicals

Plant chemicals in cerassee include: steroidal saponins, charantins; alkaloids; glycosides; carotenoids; flavonoids; coumarins; phenols; steroids

Other Uses

The cerassee fruits can be eaten when ripe. The green fruits are used for culinary purposes.

Caution!

Cerassee should not be used by people who are on drugs for cholesterol or diabetes without the supervision of a health practitioner. Cerassee should not to be used when pregnant.

CHRISTMAS CANDLESTICK – Leonotis nepetifolia – Lamiaceae

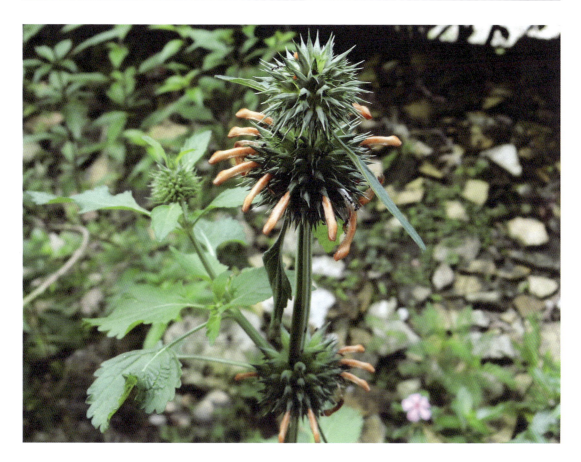

Other Names: Bald Head; Ball Bush; Lion's Ear; Klip Dagga; Shandilay; Gros Bouton; Bird Honey; Shandileer; Knod Grass; Gathivan; Cordao de Frade; Go Ponpon; Bradi-bita; Devil's Pincushion

Brief Description

Christmas candlestick is an aromatic, annual herb which grows up to two metres in height. It is native to Africa but now grows in most tropical and sub-tropical regions. The slender stems are distinctly four-sided and the hairy, heart-shaped leaves are larger on the lower part of the stem and get smaller towards the top of the plant. Bright orange flowers bear from the spiky green clusters that form at intervals along the upper portion of the plant.

Parts Used: Leaves; Flowers; Roots; Stems

Traditional Uses

In Jamaica, christmas candlestick was traditionally used for fevers, skin problems and as an abortifacient. Babies with prickly heat rash were bathed in a decoction of the leaves. Christmas candlestick is used in Trinidad for a wide variety of health conditions, including coughs, colds, asthma, stomach aches and prolapse of the womb. The leaves are also made into a salve and applied to the skin for relieving the itching caused by eczema.

Christmas candlestick is common in Brazil, where the plant is regarded as an effective treatment for sinusitis, bronchitis, stomach problems and for poor circulation. In India, all parts of the plant are used for conditions from burns, breast swelling, joint pains, malaria and ringworm to diabetes, jaundice and kidney problems.

In Africa, christmas candlestick is used wherever it grows for many different health problems. It is regarded as being effective for treating epilepsy, diarrhoea and menstrual pain, fever, swellings, skin disorders and gastro-intestinal disorders. The Khoikhoi people of the Cape region of South Africa smoked the leaves and flowers of the christmas candlestick, in much the same way as Europeans smoked tobacco, but also used it for medicinal purposes. It is still used in South Africa for asthma, epilepsy, menstrual pain and as an abortifacient. In Rwanda, a leaf decoction is traditionally used for pneumonia and some sexually transmitted infections.

Modern Research and Uses

Research into the health benefits of christmas candlestick has given credibility to some of the traditional uses of the plant and has also indicated new and potentially significant areas for further research. A number of laboratory trials, in vitro, have reported that christmas candlestick has antioxidant and anti-diabetic properties and has demonstrated effects on some cancer cell lines. Other studies indicate that the active compounds in christmas candlestick have anti-convulsant activity, which lends credence to traditional use of the herb for epilepsy. Research has also indicated wound-healing, anti-inflammatory and analgesic properties.

Recent research suggests that christmas candlestick could be useful as a preventative agent for liver disorders and is also effective in cases of diarrhoea. Studies relating to anti-microbial activity have had mixed results, with one concluding that the leaves were not very effective against some bacteria and fungi. Another study, however, reported potent antibacterial activity against bacteria including Staphylococcus aureus and Helicobacter pylori. The differences in results could be due to variations in the quality of the plant material, but this also indicates that more research should be undertaken on the different parts of christmas candlestick, as there is enough evidence that the plant has good pharmacological potential that needs to be explored more thoroughly.

Plant Chemicals

Plant chemicals in christmas candlestick include: alkaloids; flavonoids; phenols; glycosides; terpenoids; steroids; essential oils.

Other Uses

The dried leaves and flowers of the christmas candlestick are smoked for its calming effects, euphoric and psychoactive properties. The herb is currently marketed on the internet as a legal substitute for marijuana. Christmas candlestick has long been regarded as a 'holy herb' by practitioners of the Condomble religion in Brazil as well as the Winti religion in Surinam.

DANDELION – Cassia occidentalis (syn. Senna occidentalis) – Caesalpiniaceae

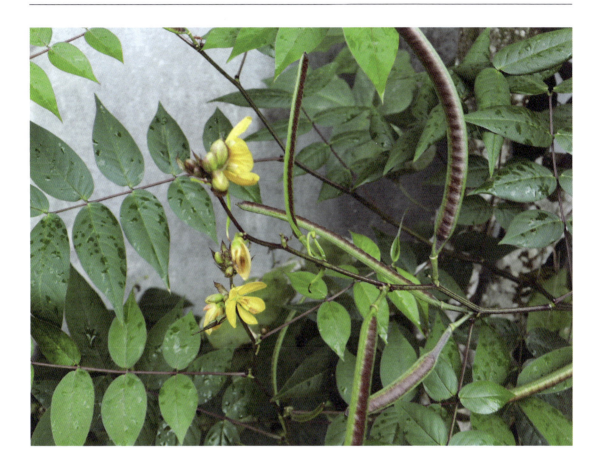

Other Names: Wild Coffee; Piss-a-bed; Negro Coffee; Fedogoso; Balatong Aso; Z'Herbe Piantes; Sanga; Coffee Senna; Mwengia; Coffee Weed; Abo Ere; Mogdad Coffee

Brief Description

Dandelion is not the 'dandelion' usually referred to in Western herbal systems. This shrub is native to South America but now grows in many tropical parts of the world. Dandelion grows up to three metres in height and has compound leaves. The plant has clusters of small yellow flowers that bear thin pods which contain small seeds.

Parts Used: Leaves; Roots; Seeds; Flowers

Traditional Uses

Dandelion has a good reputation as a healing herb wherever it grows. In Jamaica, the seeds are the most popularly used part of the plant and are roasted, ground and brewed into a coffee-like beverage that is mainly used for colds, kidney problems, as a liver tonic and for shortness of breath. It is also used to prevent bed-wetting and other bladder problems. Dandelion leaves are used externally for ringworm and other skin conditions. The roots are decocted to treat jaundice and liver disorders. Dandelion is used for similar purposes in Africa; in Ghana, dandelion is said to be good for kidney problems, stomach disorders and for blood in the urine.

In the Eastern Caribbean, the flowers and roots are used for colds and stomach disorders and the roots are soaked in warm water and used externally for skin disorders and swelling in the legs. In South America, it is valued for its liver-toning activity and used to detoxify the body, cleanse the blood and enhance immune function. Dandelion is used in Brazil to treat menstrual and urinary tract disorders and as a general tonic for weakness. In many South and Central American countries, the leaves are crushed and the juice applied to the skin to treat many types of skin problems. The tea is used internally to treat colic and intestinal parasites or applied as a poultice to relieve swellings, treat abscesses or for inflamed joints.

Modern Research and Uses

Most of the research that has been carried out on dandelion has focused on the effects of the herb on the liver and on the immune system. These studies, done on rats and other animals, have confirmed that the active plant chemicals in dandelion are effective in cases of hepatitis and other liver disorders. These chemicals also have a beneficial effect on the immune system and recent in vitro laboratory tests, an aqueous extract of dandelion demonstrated cytotoxic effects against several human cancer cell lines.

Other trials on animals have shown anti-inflammatory, anti-spasmodic and hypotensive activity. Dandelion leaf extracts were reported to be anti-diabetic in tests carried out on mice, and the plant has also exhibited anti-microbial, anti-fungal, and anti-malarial properties. Modern research has confirmed many of the traditional uses of dandelion, but more research is required.

Plant Chemicals

Plant Chemicals in dandelion include: alkaloids; saponins; terpenoids; phenols; steroids; essential oils; tannins; glycosides; flavonoids.

> **Caution!**
>
> There have been reports of toxicity in the seeds, especially when used for extended periods or in large quantities. The leaves and roots, which are effective, have lower toxicity but should still be used with caution by people with pre-existing health problems and under guidance of a health practitioner.

DONKEY PEEPEE TREE – Spathodea campanulata – Bignoniaceae

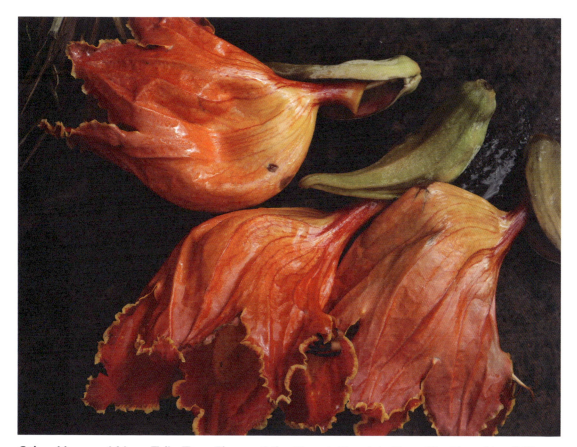

Other Names: African Tulip Tree; Flame of the Forest; Fountain Tree; Fire Tree; Nandi Flame; Squirt Tree; Amapola; Sirit-Sirit; Fire Bell; Fireball; Kibobakasi

Brief Description

Donkey peepee tree is native to the forests of Africa, but now grows in many tropical and sub-tropical regions of the world. The tree can reach a height of more than 20 metres, with dense, compound leaves made up of 5-8 pairs of pointed leaflets. The brown, unopened flower buds are filled with a liquid, which is sometimes squirted by children. The Jamaican common name reflects what people think the liquid smells like.

The large, showy flowers are up to ten centimetres long and five centimetres wide and are usually a bright orange to scarlet colour. The fruit of the tree, which is hard and brown when ripe, is about 20 centimetres long and breaks open when it falls from the tree. Each fruit contains many small seeds, which are about two centimetres wide with transparent wings.

Parts Used: Bark; Leaves; Flowers; Root Bark

Traditional Uses

The only part of the donkey peepee tree that is used for medicinal purposes in Jamaica is the liquid from the buds, which is said to be effective in treating eye infections. In other parts of the world, almost all parts of the tree are utilised for a wide variety of ailments. In Africa, donkey peepee remains a popular traditional herb. In Ghana, the stem bark is used for stomach aches, peptic ulcers and toothaches. In other West African countries, a decoction of the donkey peepee tree bark is taken for various stomach problems as well as for fevers and malaria, whereas in Rwanda, a decoction of the stem bark is considered effective for diabetes.

The flowers and leaves are applied traditionally to wounds and burns and hard-to-heal sores. The flowers are also used for inflammation of the genito-urinary tract and as a diuretic. In Southern Nigeria, the leaves are regarded as an effective treatment for painful, inflammatory conditions and for convulsions. In the Indian Ayurvedic healing system, donkey peepee is used for kidney disease. In Brazil, the leaves and flowers are also used for kidney problems and for inflammation of the urethra; the stem bark is used for stomach problems, including diarrhoea, and externally for fungal skin infections and herpes.

Modern Research and Uses

The wide variety of traditional medicinal uses for the donkey peepee tree has pointed the way for the studies carried out on the different parts of the tree. In three studies, in vitro tests on the effectiveness of the bark, leaves and flowers of the donkey peepee tree reported positive results on bacteria, including Staphylococcus aureus, E. coli and salmonella.

In a study on mice, a methanol extract of dried powdered bark made into an ointment was used to promote healing in burns. In another study using laboratory rats, a cream made from the dried stem bark of the donkey peepee tree demonstrated wound healing activity comparable to a commercially available antibiotic cream.

Studies undertaken on donkey peepee leaf extracts reported anti-convulsant, antioxidant and anti-malarial activity. Other studies also reported that leaf extracts were analgesic and anti-inflammatory. In an experiment with mice, the stem bark decoction reduced blood glucose levels, although not significantly.

An ethanol extract of donkey peepee tree bark demonstrated protective effects on the kidneys of laboratory rats. In another study, an aqueous extract of the tree's stem bark showed protective effects on the livers of rats.

Although there needs to be further research on the medicinal potential of donkey peepee tree, the studies so far have provided some scientific basis for many of the traditional uses of the various parts of this wild tree.

Plant Chemicals

Plant chemicals in the donkey peepee tree include: steroids; phenols; flavonoids; tannins; terpenoids; glycosides.

Other Uses

The seeds of the fruits are reported to be edible, but care should be taken as hunters in parts of West Africa are said to extract a poison for arrows from the boiled seeds.

In Singapore, the soft wood of the tree is used to make paper, and in some parts of Africa, the wood is used to make drums. The flowers make a lovely pastel dye for natural fabrics, especially silk. The donkey peepee tree is one of the most attractive ornamental trees, while providing other ecological and economic benefits.

FATTEN BARROW – Synedrella nodiflora – Asteraceae

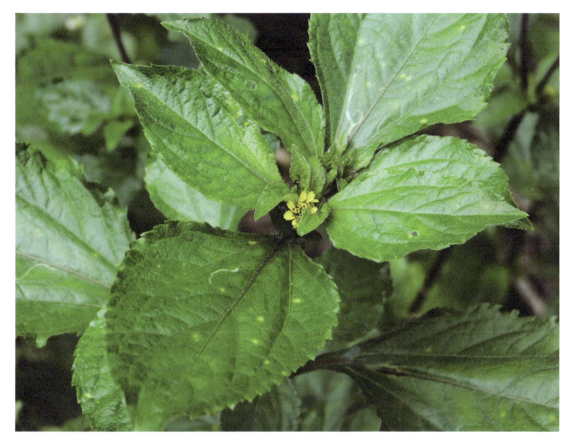

Other Names: Cinderella Bush; Porter Bush; Node Weed; Pig Weed; Herbe a Feu; Kimkim; Barbatana; Feuilles Depot; Cerbatana; Awaro Ona

Brief Description

Fatten Barrow is native to the Americas and the West Indies but is now distributed throughout tropical parts of the world. It is an erect herb, 30-80 centimetres in height, with woody stems and swollen nodes. The oval leaves are 4-9 centimetres in length, with the upper leaves being shorter than the lower ones. The bright yellow flowers bear at the intersection of the nodes and leaves.

Parts Used: Whole Plant

Traditional Uses

Fatten Barrow is traditionally used in Jamaica for colds but is said to be effective for cold sores and other skin infections. In the Eastern Caribbean, it is used for colds, coughs and fever and in Haiti for wounds and skin problems. Fatten barrow is more widely used medicinally in various parts of Africa. In Nigeria, the herb is used for wounds, to stop bleeding and for heart problems. In Ghana, the whole plant is boiled and drunk for epilepsy and is said to be an effective laxative.

In Indonesia, Malaysia and other parts of Asia, a poultice of fatten barrow leaves is applied to swollen and rheumatic joints for relief. The herb is also said to be useful for headaches and stomach problems and the leaf juice for earaches.

Modern Research and Uses

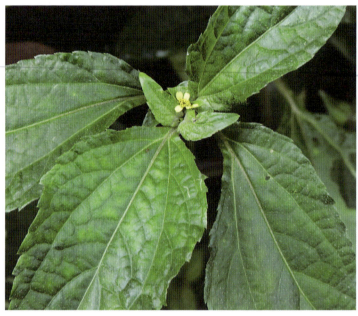

Recent research on fatten barrow has focused on some of the traditional uses of the herb. In one study in Ghana, an ethanol-and-water extract of fatten barrow plants demonstrated significant anti-convulsant effects in rats with chemically induced seizures. The specific plant chemicals that are responsible for these effects have not yet been identified.

Other studies have indicated that fatten barrow has analgesic properties and affects the central nervous system. In fact, in one animal study, an extract of the herb demonstrated protective effects on the brain after an ischaemic stroke.

Research has shown that fatten barrow has a wide variety of medicinal properties. It is anti-inflammatory, anti-microbial, antioxidant, anti-fungal, hypoglycaemic and anti-diarrhoeal. The plant has the potential to be a source of a range of pharmacological products and therefore requires further research.

Plant Chemicals

Plant chemicals in fatten barrow include: flavonoids; alkaloids; glycosides; tannins; terpenoids; phenols.

Other Uses

Young fatten barrow leaves are used as a vegetable in some countries in Southeast Asia, particularly Indonesia. In some rural parts of Jamaica, it is used as a substitute for callaloo or Indian kale in pepperpot soup.

Methanol extracts of the entire plant are said to be effective as an insecticide and larvicide, so might be useful in agriculture and for mosquito eradication. In Bangladesh, fatten barrow is used to treat cattle for swollen stomachs. Fatten barrow is also used as animal fodder in many countries and was popular as rabbit food in Jamaica.

FOUR O' CLOCK – *Mirabilis jalapa* – Nyctaginaceae

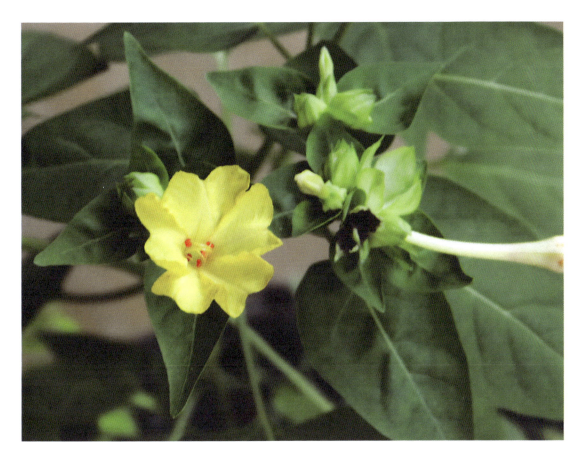

Other Names: Beauty of the Night; Belle de Nuit; Clavilla; Jalap; Marvel of Peru; Maravilla; Gulabbas; A las Quatro; Morning Rose; Buenas Tardes

Brief Description

The four o'clock plant is a perennial plant that is said to have originated in Peru but now grows in many tropical and sub-tropical parts of the world. The herb is erect, growing up to one metre high, with a number of branches which have swollen nodes at the joints. The plant bears flowers that can be white, yellow, pink, red, purple or multi-coloured and have a sweet fragrance. In fact, flowers of different colours can grow on the same plant and bloom from late afternoon, hence the name four o'clock, until early morning. When the flowers have dried up, they leave distinct black seeds. The root of the four o'clock plant is a tuber which can be up to 20 centimetres long.

Parts used: Leaves; Flowers; Root/Tuber

Traditional Uses

Four o' clock has a long history of traditional use as a healing herb in most of the countries where the plant grows. In Jamaica, it is primarily used as a healing bath for fevers, as a tea for colds and as a laxative. In other parts of the Caribbean, four o' clock is traditionally used for a range of health problems, including intestinal parasites, liver problems, menstrual irregularities, muscle pains and tumours.

Four o' clock is still a popular healing herb in South and Central America. In Mexico, a decoction of the whole plant is drunk for colic, diarrhoea, dysentery and vaginal discharge, and the leaves are rubbed and applied topically for bee and scorpion stings. In Brazil, the leaves are used to treat painful and inflammatory conditions; the leaves and flowers are combined to treat eczema and skin infections. In Peru, where four o' clock is native, the juice of the flowers is applied to herpes lesions and for earaches, while the tuber is used as a diuretic and laxative.

In Chinese traditional medicine, four o' clock is recommended for treating diabetes, and in Indonesia and India, the crushed leaves are applied to boils, abscesses and wounds. The leaf juice is also used as a douche for vaginal discharge and infections.

Modern Research and Uses

Most of the research on the four o' clock plant has been carried out over the past ten years. To date, the findings have provided some scientific support for many of the traditional uses and have pointed the way to novel applications.

A number of studies, in vitro, reported significant anti-microbial and antibacterial activity of different parts of the four o' clock plant. In one study, an ethanol extract of the leaves showed strong effects on some bacterial cultures but variable results on fungi. In that same study, however, extracts of four o'clock leaves had high levels of antioxidant and free radical scavenging activity, which suggests the effectiveness of this herb in treating degenerative conditions.

Other experiments on mice and rabbits have confirmed four o'clock's pain-relieving and anti-spasmodic properties. In a recent study, an extract of the aerial parts of the plant proved to be very effective in destroying an earthworm that causes intestinal infestation. Although the extract took longer to paralyse and kill the worm, it performed comparable to Albendazole: a commercially available anthelmintic. Animal studies have also demonstrated anti-diabetic and anti-haemorrhagic properties.

An area of research that is now developing around four o'clock is the usefulness of extracts of the seeds and root/tubers. There are ongoing debates as to the level of toxicity in the seeds and tubers, which have been used traditionally both internally and externally. It might be best to avoid ingesting the seeds and to exercise caution when using the root (see below). There is increasing evidence that phytochemicals extracted from the seeds have medicinal potential for a variety of diseases including cancer and HIV.

A recent study in Nigeria, using mice, found that leaf extracts of the four o'clock plant had significant anti-malarial effects, establishing a rationale for traditional use of the plant for this purpose there.

The range of health conditions that can be treated by the different parts of the four o'clock plant indicates that further studies need to be undertaken to refine current understanding of the active chemicals in the plant and how these can be utilised effectively.

Plant Chemicals

Plant chemicals in four o' clock include: proteins; glycosides; flavonoids; saponins; betalains; rotenoids; phenols; alkaloids; steroids.

Other Uses

An edible dye from the flowers of the four o'clock plant is used as a colourant in cosmetics, cakes and other confectionery. In Malaysia, China and Japan, the powdered seeds are used as a cosmetic powder, and the root powder mixed with sandalwood is also used for this purpose.

The mirabilis antiviral proteins (MAPs) in four o'clock have been patented for use in protecting commercial crops such as potato, tobacco and corn from various plant viruses.

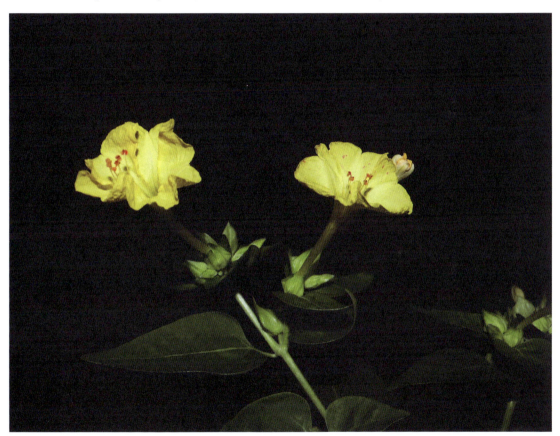

Caution!

There are high levels of peptides in the seeds of the four o'clock plant that are similar to neuro-toxic substances such as ricin. Although similar, they are only a fraction of the toxicity of other peptides; however, it is advisable not to use the seeds internally, unless under the guidance of a qualified practitioner. The roots should be used with caution internally. Four o'clock also contains other chemicals which are known to stimulate the uterus so should not be used in pregnancy.

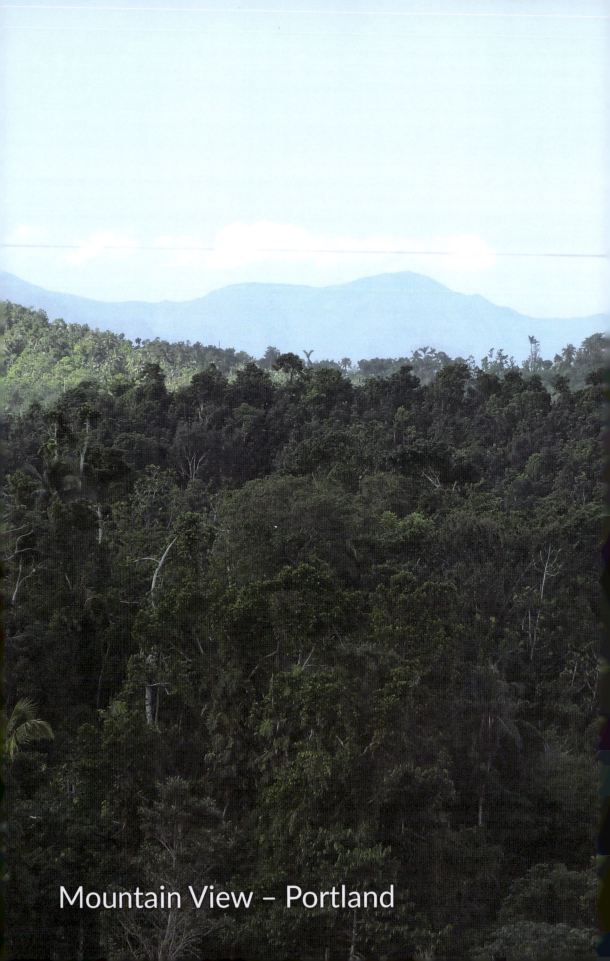

Mountain View – Portland

GANJA – Cannabis sativa / Cannabis indica – Cannabaceae

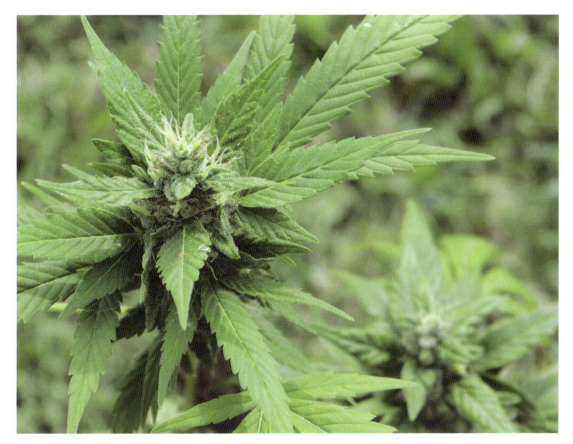

Other Names: Marijuana; Grass; Herbs; Cannabis; Bhang; Dagga; Weed

Brief Description

Grown in many parts of the world, ganja is a bushy shrub which can grow up to four metres in height. It is grown legally for use as a fibre (hemp) and for the seeds. It is also grown illegally for the flowering tops of the female plants, which are mainly used as a recreational substance.

Parts Used: Leaves; Roots; Flowering Tops; Oil

Traditional Uses

Ganja has a very long history in herbal healing, dating back to ancient Egypt, where it was used to treat inflammation of the eye. It is used in traditional Indian and Chinese medicine for congestion, rheumatism, malaria and constipation and as a local anaesthetic. In the nineteenth century, ganja was commonly used as a painkiller, particularly for menstrual pain and cramps.

In Jamaica, ganja is traditionally used to treat colds, flu, asthma, stomach problems and to improve eyesight. Oil- or alcohol-based extracts and infusions are used in many traditional herbal remedies. Ganja is soaked in rum with ginger, garlic and pimento and taken internally to treat diarrhoea and externally for relieving joint pains. In Ghana, ganja is also used for pain relief, as a local anaesthetic and in aphrodisiac concoctions.

Modern Research and Uses

There have been numerous studies of ganja, many of which focused on the recreational use of the plant in relation to its legal status and effects on the health of users. Recently, there has been more research on the medicinal properties of ganja and the possible uses of the herb to treat a variety of health conditions.

Research in Jamaica confirmed that ganja is effective in treating eye conditions, in particular glaucoma, and an extract of ganja (Cannasol) is commercially available to treat this condition. Another medicine made from ganja (Asmasol), has been patented for the treatment of asthma.

Ganja's traditional use as a pain reliever has been confirmed by recent research, which shows that it can be as effective as codeine. It is also reported to have sedative, anti-inflammatory and anti-emetic properties, making it effective for nausea, especially for people receiving chemotherapy. Ganja is now being used with good results in relieving the symptoms of multiple sclerosis and epilepsy, treating people with spinal cord injuries and for loss of appetite. The tetrahydrocannabinol (THC) content in ganja has also been proven to be effective in treating people with sleep disorders, including sleep apnoea.

In recent years, there have been more studies into what is termed 'medical marijuana', and there is now enough evidence for the use of ganja to treat a variety of health conditions. The Federal Drugs Agency (FDA) has already approved a synthetic THC pill called Marinol to treat nausea. Much of the current debate in medical circles centres on the use of one of the over 60 cannabinoids in ganja: cannabidiol, or CBD. CBD does not have the same psychoactive properties as THC and is reported to be very effective in treating a range of disorders, including anxiety, depression, epilepsy and schizophrenia. There are reports that clinical trials are underway to explore the effects of CBD on breast cancer as well as on a number of degenerative illnesses.

Plant Chemicals

Plant chemicals in ganja include: cannabinoids; terpenoids; steroids; flavonoids; phenols; alkaloids; essential oils.

Other Uses

The dried leaves and flowering tops are smoked recreationally in many countries. Rastafarians regard ganja as a sacred herb with the power to improve meditation and understanding. There has been increasing production of hemp as a viable economic crop with a wide variety of uses and applications. Hemp seed is rich in omega oils and many other essential nutrients. Bio-industries in countries like Switzerland have developed a number of health, clothing, beauty and medicinal products from hemp and hemp seed for export and local consumption.

Caution!

Smoking ganja, as with any form of smoking, can lead to lung and other bronchial and respiratory problems. Those concerned about smoking can ingest ganja in various ways, such as cooking, baking and using extracts that are oil or alcohol based. Some studies have, however, reported that regular, long-term use can lead to psychiatric, psychological and neurological problems.

It is illegal to grow or possess ganja in Jamaica and in many countries.

GUACO – *Mikania micrantha* – Asteraceae

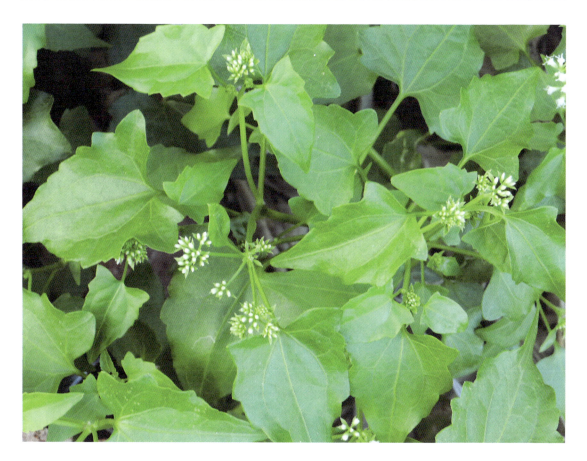

Other Names: Gwaco; Quaco; Snake Vine; Cepu; Bitter Vine; Climbing Hempweed; Mile-a-Minute; Bitter Tally; Kacho

Brief Description

Guaco is a common, spreading, tropical vine that can be found in many parts of Central and South America, the Caribbean, Africa and Southeast Asia. The vine is more succulent than woody with heart-shaped leaves. The vine bears whitish or yellowish flowers, which have a pleasant smell.

Parts Used: Leaves; Vines; Roots

Traditional Uses

In Jamaica, guaco is traditionally used for colds and drunk either as an infusion or as a fresh-leaf juice for this purpose. Externally, it is used for skin problems such as sores, boils, rashes and severe itching. A decoction is made for chest and stomach pains and for diarrhoea. In Jamaica, a heated pad of guaco leaves is applied to joints to relieve pain from rheumatism and gout. The plant is used in similar ways in other parts of the Caribbean.

In South America and parts of Africa, guaco is used for snake, scorpion and dog bites, sexually transmitted infections, asthma and all kinds of respiratory problems, including bronchitis. In

Brazil, a cough syrup made from guaco is still used in many homes. Guaco is also reputed to be effective for eczema and wounds. In Ghana, it is used for fevers, eye problems, cholera and for snake and other bites as in South America.

Modern Research and Uses

Many of the traditional uses of guaco have been validated by the few studies that have been carried out on the plant. In Brazil, the use of guaco for respiratory problems was reported more than 60 years ago, and human trials confirmed these findings over 20 years ago. More recent research has demonstrated that guaco has anti-fungal, anti-inflammatory, anti-spasmodic and anti-protozoal properties.

Research at the University of the West Indies (UWI) in Jamaica reported that guaco was effective against E. coli, Staphylococcus aureus and streptococcus aureus bacteria. The study also found that guaco has hypoglycaemic activity but that it was short-lived. Guaco's anti-microbial properties have been confirmed in other studies, with suggestions that the active plant chemicals should be identified and developed for pharmaceutical production and application.

Methanol extracts of guaco root were reported to have significant effects on mice with liver disease, inflammation and pain. Findings from other research indicate that sesquiterpene dilactones are responsible for the plant's anti-inflammatory and anti-carcinogenic properties.

Emerging research on guaco points to the fact that this plant has the potential to be effective against a range of diseases and health conditions, but further research is needed.

Plant Chemicals

The plant chemicals in guaco include: terpenoids; coumarins; glycosides; phenols; tannins; flavonoids; steroids.

Caution!

For people taking blood-thinning drugs, it is important to seek advice from a health professional before using guaco internally due to its high coumarin content.

GUAVA – Psidium guajava – Myrtaceae

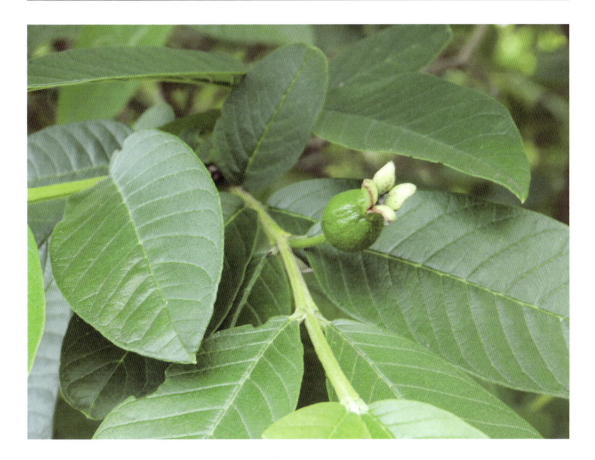

Other Names: Guayabo; Gouyave; Jambu; Bayabas; Koyya; Aduaba

Brief Description

Guava is a common tree in the tropics, which can grow up to ten metres in height. It is native to the Americas, but has now spread to other tropical and sub-tropical regions. It has a distinctive bark that is light coloured and peels to show the layer beneath, similar to another member of that genus, pimento. Guava has rough, light-green leaves and the tree bears small white flowers. The fruit of the guava varies according to growing conditions and variety, but can be as big as an orange, with numerous small seeds.

Parts Used: Fruits; Leaves; Buds; Bark; Seeds; Twigs

Traditional Uses

Guava leaves are used traditionally in Jamaica for diarrhoea and for bathing wounds. Similar use is made of guava in the rest of the Caribbean, where the leaves and buds are used for diarrhoea, dysentery and stomach aches. In Ghana, guava is also used for stomach problems, diarrhoea and coughs; the leaves are chewed for toothache.

In the Canary Islands, guava is used for vomiting and nausea as well as for diarrhoea. In South and Central America, the leaves and bark of the guava tree are used to treat dysentery and diarrhoea and also in a gargle for sore throats. A decoction of guava leaves is taken internally to reduce vaginal discharges and relieve menstrual pain. It can also be applied topically for skin ulcers and vaginal irritation. Guava leaves are boiled with fever grass, ginger and passion flower leaves to make a syrup for colds and coughs. Guava pulp and leaves are used for gastro-intestinal illnesses in Southeast Asian countries. There is a lot of similarity in the use of guava, wherever it grows, which suggests that it is effective against those conditions.

Modern Research and Uses

Modern research has concluded that guava's effectiveness in treating dysentery and diarrhoea is due mainly to its active plant chemicals, particularly the high content of quercetins. A standardised extract is now available, and a clinical trial in humans has shown that both the guava leaf extract and the juice are effective in treating rotavirus enteritis in infants.

Guava has demonstrated antibacterial, anti-fungal, anti-amoebic, anti-spasmodic and anti-malarial properties. Laboratory tests have shown that extracts of guava leaves and bark are toxic to a number of bacteria. These properties might explain why guava has been used traditionally for skin infections, wounds and ulcers as well as its effectiveness in treating respiratory problems.

Animal trials have indicated that the leaf extracts might be useful in treating irregular heartbeat. Other research has suggested that guava could also be effective in reducing cardiovascular risk factors such as high blood pressure, blood sugar and cholesterol. A study in humans reported that after using guava for 12 weeks, there was a significant reduction in their blood pressure, cholesterol and triglycerides, which are beneficial to overall cardiovascular health.

Animal studies have shown that methanol extracts of the leaves have anti-inflammatory and analgesic properties, which again validate the traditional use of guava leaves for toothache and menstrual pain. Yet another study has indicated that guava can be effective as a central nervous system depressant, which can help with sleeplessness and anxiety.

Recent research has reported that a hexane extract of guava leaves had cytotoxic effects on two cancer lines and indicated that further studies need to be carried out to find which compounds in guava leaves are responsible for this effect.

Plant Chemicals

The plant chemicals in guava include: tannins; terpenoids; phenols; carotenoids; flavonoids; phenylpropanoids; saponins; glycosides.

Other Uses

Guava is rich in vitamins C and A. The fruits are used both domestically and commercially to make preserves, jams and a local Caribbean delicacy called 'guava cheese'. Guava is also made into drinks sometimes in combination with other fruits.

> **Caution!**
>
> Due to evidence of guava's effects on cardiovascular health, people taking medications for blood pressure, diabetes or heart problems should use guava with care over long periods of time, in case of any adverse interaction with prescribed medicines.

GUINEA HEN WEED – *Petiveria alliacea* – Phytolaccaceae

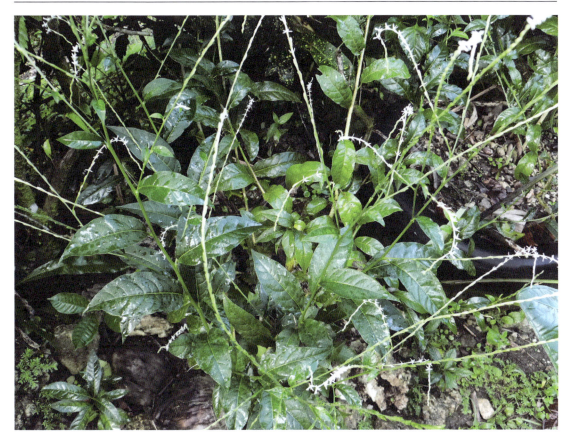

Other Names: Strong Man Weed; Conga Root; Gully Root; Kojo Root; Garlic Weed; Mawi Pouwi; Anamu; Mapurite; Danday; Kudjuruk; Arada

Brief Description

Guinea hen weed is native to the tropical Americas and now grows in other tropical parts of the world. The plant has a slender stem and thick tap root, with pointed leaves up to 15 centimetres long. Tiny greenish-white flowers bear on spikes which can be seen all year round. The herb is distinguished by its strong, garlic-like smell.

Parts Used: Leaves; Roots; Whole Plant

Traditional Uses

Guinea hen weed is used traditionally in Jamaica to treat fever, headache and general pains, fits, hysteria, sinus and flu. It is also regarded as an antidote for poisoning. In the Eastern Caribbean, the leaves are rubbed and inhaled for headaches and combined with fits weed to treat fevers. Guinea hen weed is also steeped in rum and drunk as an aphrodisiac or applied topically to skin eruptions. In Cuba, herbalists decoct the whole plant and use it to treat cancer, diabetes and inflammatory conditions.

Guinea hen weed has a long history in herbal medicine in all of the countries where it grows. Throughout Central America, women use guinea hen weed to relieve birthing pains and facilitate easy childbirth as well as to induce abortions. In Guatemalan herbal medicine, the plant is made into a decoction and taken internally for sluggish digestion and flatulence. A leaf decoction is also used topically as an analgesic for muscular pain and for skin diseases. Guinea hen weed is still used widely in South and Central America, where it is commonly sold in big cities and towns as a natural remedy for colds, coughs, influenza, respiratory and pulmonary infections and to support the immune system.

Modern Research and Uses

Much of the research conducted on guinea hen weed has focused on the anti-cancerous and anti-tumorous activity of extracts as well as its effect on stimulating the immune system. Dibenzyl trisulphide (DTS) has been identified as the key compound in guinea hen weed that might be responsible for the plant's effect on tumours. A recent study indicates that it activates bone marrow, is anti-microbial and anti-inflammatory. There has also been an experimental study looking at the mechanism by which benzyl trisulphide extracted from guinea hen weed can suppress the immune system in order to treat people with lupus and potentially other autoimmune conditions. Other studies on mice confirm that extracts of guinea hen leaves have pain-relieving properties, which, again, validate some of the traditional uses for this herb.

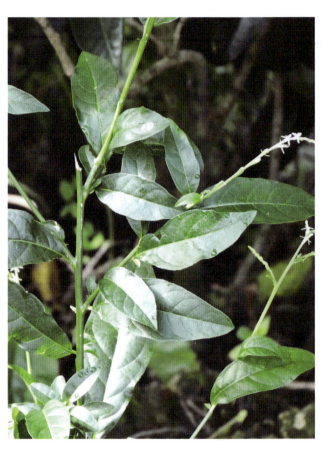

A recent laboratory study in Cuba found that a hydro-ethanol extract of guinea hen weed leaves was able to inhibit the growth of candida cells. It has also recently been reported that guinea hen weed can be effective in treating cystitis, prostatitis and potentially be an adjunct therapy for prostate cancer.

Plant Chemicals

Plant chemicals in guinea hen weed include: flavonoids; terpenoids; steroids; sulphur compounds; coumarins; phenols; saponins; allantoin; tannins; squalene; allantoin.

Caution!

Guinea hen weed should not be used by pregnant women. Anyone with diabetes or a heart condition should not use guinea hen weed without medical supervision

HOG PLUM – Spondias mombin – Anacardiaceae

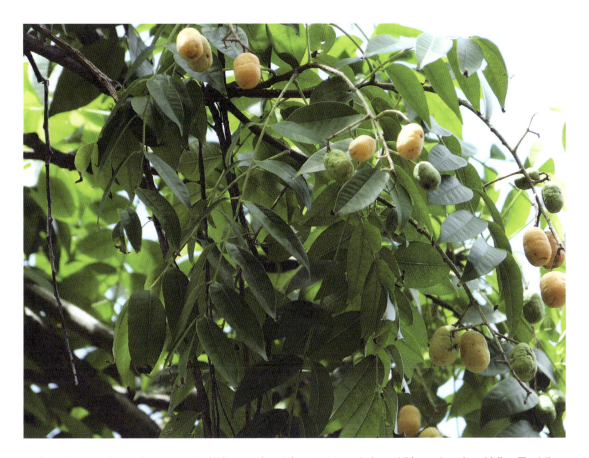

Other Names: Java Plum; Tropical Plum; Jobo; Ubos; Mope; Ashanti Plum; Ataaba; Akika; Tapiriba; Acaiba; Prune Mombin

Brief Description

Hog plum grows in many tropical areas. The erect tree can reach a height of 20 metres. The trunk has deep incisions in the bark that produce a brown resin. Before the tree starts to flower, it strips itself of most of the leaves and bears small, fragrant, whitish flowers. The small green fruits bear in clusters, turning yellow when ripe.

Parts Used: Buds; Roots; Bark; Leaves; Fruits

Traditional Uses

Hog plum is not widely used now as a healing herb in Jamaica, but the bark and leaves used to be given as a tea to relieve swellings and the buds chewed or made into a tea for colds, coughs, constipation and tapeworm. In the Eastern Caribbean, a decoction of hog plum bud, roots and bark was traditionally used to treat gonorrhoea, diarrhoea, dysentery, and as an eyewash. A poultice from hog plum leaves is still used to treat sores. In Suriname, hog plum is used in similar ways as in the Caribbean.

Hog plum leaves and bark are still widely used in South America for female reproductive problems. The leaves are valued by traditional midwives, particularly for treating bleeding in childbirth and excessive menstrual bleeding. A decoction of hog plum leaves and bark can be effective when used topically for a range of skin conditions, including ulcers, rashes, psoriasis and wounds. The bark extract is thought by some traditional healers to prevent and treat malaria. In Ghana, hog plum is used for a wide variety of health conditions, including coughs, fever, eye problems, as a diuretic and to treat stomach aches and uterine cancer.

Modern Research and Uses

Recent research in Nigeria has suggested a wide range of uses for hog plum. It has anti-microbial effects that are reported to be as broad spectrum as ampicillin and gentamicin. In laboratory tests, an extract of hog plum leaves was effective against the bacteria that cause tuberculosis, but this effect has not yet been tested on humans. Hog plum was also found to have anti-malarial properties in laboratory tests, confirming one of the traditional uses of the bark.

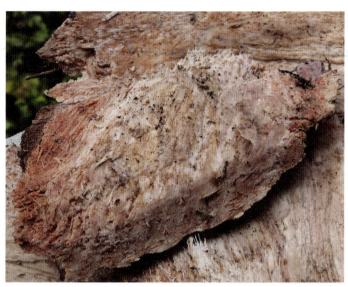

A study in rats has, for the first time, indicated that hog plum leaves have cardio-protective properties, similar to the drug Ramipril. This also suggests that hog plum could be effective in lowering blood pressure. In another study carried out in pregnant mice, hog plum was reported to have abortifacient and uterine-stimulant activity. Other studies confirm that hog plum is sedative, anthelmintic, anti-convulsant and has anti-psychotic and antioxidant effects. Much of this research lends credibility to some of the traditional uses of hog plum and highlights other effects. More research is needed to investigate the varied uses and potential of different parts of the tree.

Plant Chemicals

Plant chemicals in hog plum include: tannins; resin; saponins; flavonoids; steroids; salicylic acid derivatives; phenols; glycosides; oxalates; phytates.

Other Uses

Hog plum is usually eaten by children and in some countries made into juices, preserves and wine. The fruit is rich in vitamins B1 and C. The brown resin that comes from the bark can be used as a glue substitute.

Caution!

There is enough evidence that hog plum can stimulate the uterus so pregnant women or those trying to get pregnant should not use hog plum leaves or bark internally

---

JACK'NA BUSH – Eupatorium odoratum
(syn. Chromolaena odorata) – Asteraceae

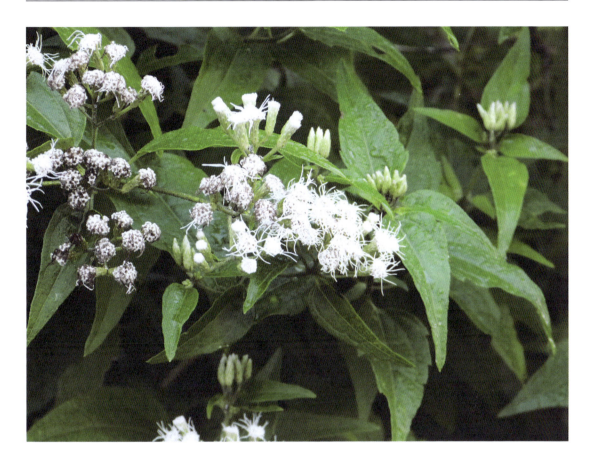

Other Names: Christmas Rose; Bitter Bush; Siam Weed; Santa Maria; Hemp Agrimony; Flewi Nwel; Hagonoy

Brief Description

Jack'na bush is a fast-growing, perennial shrub which can grow up to four metres in height and is regarded as a very invasive species. It has slightly oval leaves that have dented margins and a long tip. It is native to tropical and sub-tropical Americas, but now grows in many tropical regions. The plant has fluffy, cream flowers, which disperse on the wind when dry.

Parts Used: Leaves; Flowers

Traditional Uses

In Jamaica, an infusion of jack'na bush leaves is used for coughs, colds, flu and to treat cuts and wounds. The herb is also widely used throughout the Caribbean for coughs and colds and is boiled in milk to treat bronchitis in children.

In Nigeria and other parts of West Africa, jack'na bush is used for a wide variety of health conditions, including wounds, nosebleeds, colds and fevers, stomach disorders, skin diseases and toothache. In Southeast Asia the plant is used to reduce bleeding in wounds and to treat burns, abscesses, boils and other skin infections.

Modern Research

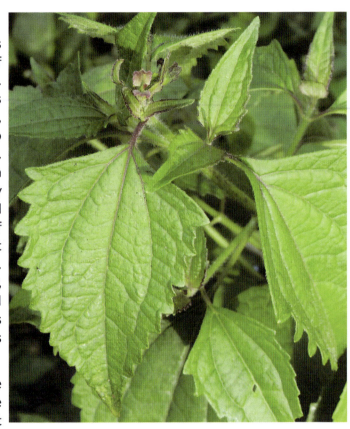

A recent study from Vietnam has confirmed the traditional use of jack'na bush to treat wounds. An extract of jack'na bush leaves lessened blood flow in wounds, promoted healing and was also effective in treating haemorrhoids. In laboratory tests, jack'na bush exhibited anti-inflammatory properties and anti-microbial activity and an alcohol extract of the leaves was effective against Staphylococcus aureus and E. coli. The aqueous extract was, however, less effective. Research at UWI also found that jack'na bush was effective against Staphylococcus aureus bacteria.

In vitro laboratory studies have reported that extracts from the plant are antioxidant and that extracts from the flowers exhibited similar antioxidant effects. Another study in mice showed that jack'na bush has diuretic effects, which could be useful for people with high blood pressure.

A recent analysis of jack'na bush leaves concluded that the plant had high mineral content, with calcium, potassium, iron, zinc, copper and magnesium, which could be utilised for health benefits.

Plant Chemicals

Plant chemicals in jack'na bush include: terpenoids; flavonoids; alkaloids; lignans; tannins; steroids; carotenoids and essential oils.

Other Uses

Based on research so far, jack'na bush has the potential to be developed into cosmetic products, especially those for skin care. A major multinational company has already filed a patent for anti-ageing creams, based on extracts from jack'na bush.

The antioxidant and nutritional content warrants further exploration as it could yield nutraceutical products. The plant is also being researched for its potential use in animal feed including chicken and egg production.

JOHN CHARLES – Hyptis verticillata – Lamiaceae

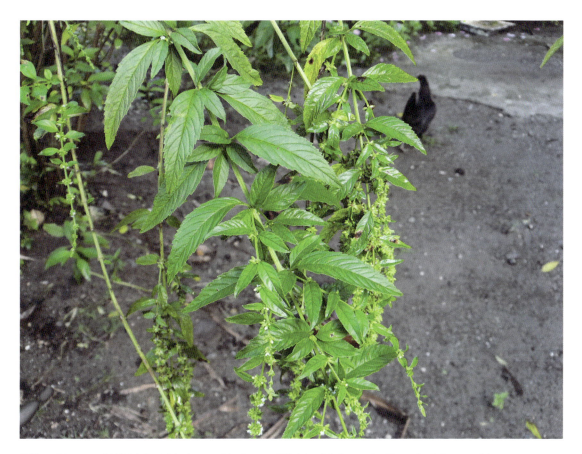

Other Names: Wild Mint, Verbena, Herbe au Diable, Malcasada Grande, Maman-Houanne

Brief Description

John charles is a native of Central America, but now grows widely in many tropical areas. The plant grows to a height of two metres, with oval, slightly toothed leaves and white flowers.

Parts Used: Leaves, Roots

Traditional Uses

In Jamaica, john charles is mainly used to treat colds and respiratory infections, skin problems like eczema and inflammatory conditions such as arthritis and gout. It was also used in herbal baths. In South and Central America, the herb is used to treat headache, backache and toothache, a variety of skin infections and also gynaecological conditions.

John charles is also used to treat headaches, stomach aches and rheumatism in Mexico, and in Haiti as a sedative and herbal bath for a variety of conditions. In Africa, the herb is used to treat colds, fevers, skin conditions and stomach disorders. The leaves are said to be more effective when they are dried.

Modern Research and Uses

Research conducted on john charles has been limited, but so far, findings have shown that this herb has many active plant chemicals that could treat a wide range of diseases and infectious organisms. Many of these confirm some of the traditional uses of the plant, particularly for skin conditions, pain relief and as an anti-inflammatory. John charles has exhibited anti-secretory properties, particularly on gastric secretions, and this could be useful in treating stomach ulcers and other stomach disorders.

Many of the plant chemicals found in john charles are unique to the herb. These phytochemicals have antibacterial, antiseptic, antiviral, anti-fungal and anti-diarrhoeal properties. A recent study confirmed that compounds in john charles have a range of activity which could be beneficial in the treatment of cancer, particularly on cancer cells that have proven resistant to a variety of drugs. Further research needs to be carried out on john charles to provide more evidence of the herb's medicinal potential.

Plant Chemicals

Plant chemicals in john charles include: terpenoids; flavonoids; phenols; alkaloids; lignans; essential oils.

Other Uses

Extracts from john charles are used to treat infections in animals and to kill ticks and other animal parasites. It was also shown to be toxic to the sweet potato pest. The leaves of john charles can be used to make aromatic and essential oils, with the potential for use in medicinal and cosmetic products.

KING OF THE FOREST – Cassia alata (syn. Senna alata) – (Caesalpiniaceae)

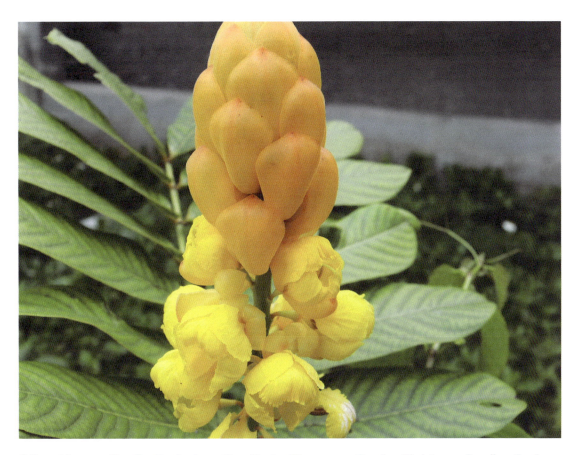

Other Names: Candle Bush; Impetigo Bush; Ringworm Cassia; Christmas Candle; Guajava; Nsempii; Seven Golden Candlesticks; Akapulko; Gelenggag; Fleur Dartres; Dartier

Brief Description

King of the forest is a shrub that is native to the tropical regions of the Americas, but is now grown in other regions of the world. King of the forest has large compound leaves, with each up to 20 centimetres long; these are coarse to the touch. The shrub bears pretty, erect, yellow flowers which look like golden candles. The tree bears fruits in the form of green pods, which hold up to 60 seeds and go brown when ripe.

Parts Used: Leaves; Roots; Bark; Fruits

Traditional Uses

A tea made from the leaves of king of the forest is traditionally used in Jamaica as a purgative; to restore the system, for high blood pressure and for skin problems. In other parts of the Caribbean, it is also used for hypertension and to treat ringworm and impetigo. The leaves are steeped in water to make a gargle, and the pulp around the seeds is used as a purgative, but the seeds are said to be poisonous.

In Suriname, the leaves are used as a laxative, but their main use is for skin problems. A decoction of the roots is also used there to treat uterine disorders. In other parts of South America, king of the forest is reputed to be effective in treating fevers, stomach problems, asthma and sexually transmitted infections such as syphilis.

King of the forest is used in parts of Africa for high blood pressure; asthma and a variety of skin conditions, including fungal infections. The plant is used in Ghana to make both a tea and a bath for women to facilitate childbirth. In Southeast Asia, it is widely used for ringworm and other fungal conditions and also as a laxative. King of the forest is traditionally used for insect bites and for sexually transmitted infections in India.

Modern Research and Uses

Research in Ghana showed that an extract from king of the forest leaves was active in lab tests against MRSA and gonorrhoea bacteria. It was shown to have anti-microbial, analgesic, and anti-inflammatory properties. Strong evidence from numerous studies confirms that king of the forest is a very effective treatment for fungal infections. A ten-year study in humans confirmed the traditional use of king of the forest to treat a fungal skin condition, tinea versicolor, commonly called 'liver spots'.

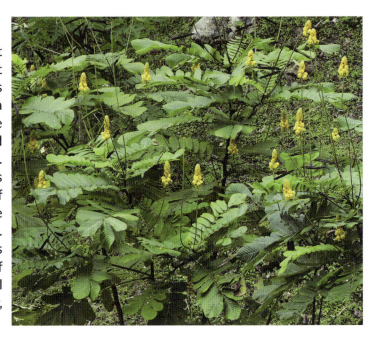

Japanese trials have confirmed the presence of an active compound which has anti-inflammatory activity. In a recent clinical trial in Thailand, the leaf extract of king of the forest was confirmed as an effective laxative. The plant was also shown to have anti-microbial activity in lab tests, inhibiting the growth of a number of bacteria. Recent reports suggest that king of the forest can help with weight loss and is potentially a source for the development of an anti-diabetic drug. Results from another study showed that a hexane extract of king of the forest has cytotoxic activity on a number of cancer cell lines. Further research is being carried out to explore the specific compounds in the plant which are responsible for these cytotoxic effects.

Plant Chemicals

Plant chemicals in king of the forest include: phenols; flavonoids; saponins; steroids; glycosides; terpenoids; essential oils.

Other Uses

In the Philippines, leaf extracts are used in the commercial production of soaps, shampoos and skin creams.

LEAF OF LIFE – Bryophyllum pinnatum (Kalanchoe pinnata) – Crassulaceae

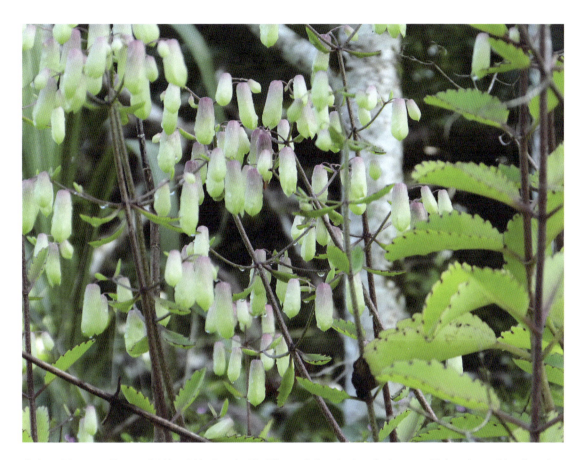

Other Names: Tree of Life; Life Leaf; Air Plant; Miracle Leaf; Aporo; Kalanchoe; Katakataka; Mother of Thousands; Cathedral Bells; Siempre Viva

Brief Description

Leaf of life is native to Africa but is now grown widely in tropical and sub-tropical areas. It is a succulent plant that grows up to 1.5 metres in height, with a reddish tinge to the stems. The leaves have indented edges, from which new plants can grow. When mature, leaf of life bears clusters of bell-shaped flowers.

Parts Used: Leaves; Stems

Traditional Uses

The juice of leaf of life is mixed with salt or honey and used in Jamaica to treat colds, coughs and bronchial problems. The leaves are softened by heat and applied to the affected part for abscesses and swollen and inflamed joints for relief. This method is also used to treat headaches. A tea made from leaf of life is reputed to be effective for hypertension and painful periods.

In the Eastern Caribbean, leaf of life is used as a tea for colds and the juice used externally for sores and headaches. It is used in Brazil for respiratory problems, such as asthma and bronchitis, and is considered an effective remedy for kidney stones and gastric ulcers. Leaf of life juice is applied topically for boils, burns, ulcers, insect bites and eye infections. In Africa, an infusion of the leaves is traditionally used as a diuretic; for earaches and eye problems. In India, leaf juice is used for asthma, as a cough suppressant and for diarrhoea.

Leaf of life is well regarded wherever it grows, and there are many similarities in the way in which the plant is used, whether in Central America or Southeast Asia. Most traditional methods require fresh plant material, which is difficult if leaf of life is not readily available. Fortunately, the plant grows easily and quickly and makes a good houseplant even in colder countries.

Modern Research and Uses

Several studies have documented leaf of life's anti-microbial, antiviral and anti-fungal activity. The plant is also said to have antihistamine and anaphylactic properties which would explain its traditional use for asthma, insect bites and stings.

In a study in Hawaii, leaf of life demonstrated noticeable effects on cancer tissue and also confirmed significant anti-microbial activity. A more recent in vitro study reported that a chloroform extract of leaf of life was effective in inhibiting the growth of human papillomavirus (HPV) and cervical cancer cells.

A study on mice in Nigeria reported that leaf of life has pain-relieving and anti-diabetic activity. Earlier research concluded that leaf of life has immunosuppressant properties that could be useful in conditions such as rheumatoid arthritis and lupus and is likely related to the plant's antihistamine and anti-inflammatory activities. A more recent study, however, suggested that leaf of life can act as an immune-modulator, selectively modifying the function of the immune system.

Leaf of life has been called a 'miracle plant', and given the wide range of applications it has, internally and externally, for so many health conditions, it is really important that there is further research into this plant.

Plant Chemicals

Plant chemicals in leaf of life include: phenols; flavonoids; terpenoids; steroids; glycosides; glucosides; saponins; carotenoids; coumarins.

Other Uses

Some types of leaf of life are available as ornamental plants. These plants are hybrids and do not have the same medicinal properties, therefore they should not be used for therapeutic purposes.

Caution!

Leaf of life contains some very potent plant chemicals and should not be used internally for extended periods, without professional advice.

MARIGOULE – Wedelia Trilobata (syn. Sphagneticola trilobata) – Asteraceae

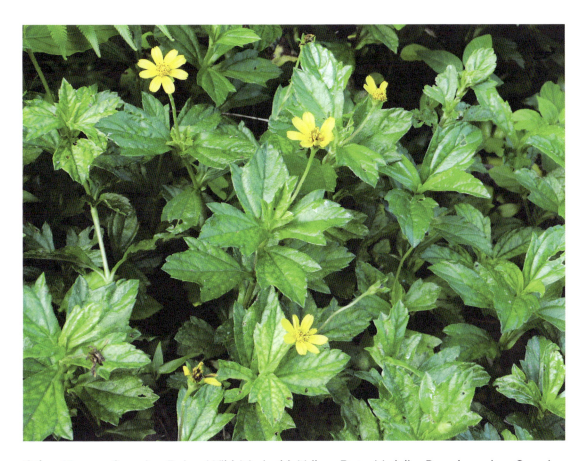

Other Names: Creeping Daisy; Wild Marigold; Yellow Dots; Vedelia; Pseudo-arnica; Creeping Oxeye; Z'herbe a Femme; Venvenn Kawayib

Brief Description

Marigoule is found in many tropical regions of the world. The plant creeps along the ground and provides thick cover that is especially useful where soil erosion is likely. The stems form roots at the nodes and the bright yellow flowers bear at the end of upright stalks. The flowers are very similar to daisies, and the shiny, bright green leaves which have three lobes give the plant its botanical name. In some countries, marigoule is regarded as an invasive species due to its extensive ground cover, which prevents other plants from growing.

Parts Used: Leaves; Stems; Flowers

Traditional Uses

Marigoule is used traditionally in Jamaica to treat colds, fevers, sores; reproductive and stomach problems. In other parts of the Caribbean, marigoule is used for female reproductive conditions such as painful periods; during and after childbirth and to clear the placenta. Marigoule is used in Trinidad and Tobago and some other Caribbean islands to improve fertility by clearing and cleansing the reproductive organs and tract.

In Central and South America, the whole plant is used to treat a wide range of health problems, including bronchitis, stings, wounds, sores, swellings, rheumatism, muscle and other cramps and backache. For these conditions, the herb is taken as an infusion, applied as a poultice or put into a bath. In Suriname, marigoule is especially prized for improving liver and digestive function and is also used to treat various genito-urinary infections. However, in Brazil, marigoule is popularly called insulina and is reputed to be effective for diabetes.

In some countries in Asia, marigoule leaves and stems are pounded and tied on to swollen, arthritic joints to relieve pain and inflammation. In Vietnam, the herb is reputed to be effective in treating fevers and malaria, and in parts of Thailand, marigoule is used for headaches and fever.

Modern Research and Use

Most of the research carried out on marigoule has tested the anti-microbial activity of the plant, and the results have varied. Earlier studies at the University of the West Indies reported that marigoule exhibited no antibacterial activity. However, recent studies have shown that extracts of the leaves, stem, root and flowers of the plant exhibited significant but varying degrees of effectiveness on a range of bacteria and fungi. The effectiveness differed according to the medium of extraction and the nature of the bacteria: there were, however, no effects on the fungi studied.

In an animal experiment, an aqueous extract of marigoule leaves not only reduced blood sugar levels but also had significant antioxidant effects that improved the overall condition of key organs, which are usually impaired as a result of diabetes. Other studies have also confirmed that marigoule has powerful free radical scavenging properties that could also be beneficial in preventing and improving other chronic health conditions, including some cancers.

Traditional uses of marigoule for pain relief and as an anti-inflammatory have been supported by recent research on the plant. What is needed now is for more studies to be undertaken to understand which plant chemicals have which effects.

Plant Chemicals

The plant chemicals in marigoule include: phenols; flavonoids; terpenoids; tannins; saponins; essential oils.

Caution!

Care should also be exercised by anyone who is taking medication for diabetes. Pregnant women should not use marigoule in the first two trimesters

---

MILK WEED – Euphorbia hirta – Euphorbiaceae

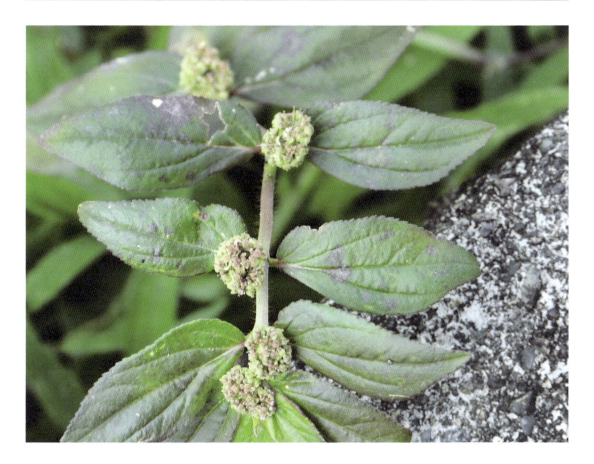

Other Names: Asthma Weed; Spurge; Pill-bearing Spurge; Wart Weed; Z'herbe Mal Nommee; Gatas-gatas, Dudhi; Cat's Hair; Snakeweed

Brief Description

Milk weed is a small, trailing weed, found in many tropical parts of the world. It often has reddish stems with greenish flowers on the stems. The plant produces a milky sap when the stems are cut.

Parts Used: Leaves; Roots; Latex (milk)

Traditional Uses

In Jamaica, milk weed is used traditionally for colds, back pain, high blood pressure and as a tonic. It is also boiled with carry mi seed to treat gonorrhoea, and the latex applied as a dressing for cuts and to remove warts. In the Eastern Caribbean, milk weed is used mainly for fevers and to promote urination as well as for asthma, bronchitis and other respiratory tract infections.

Milk weed is used traditionally in parts of Asia to treat asthma and wounds. In India, the herb is boiled to treat sexually transmitted infections and given to nursing mothers to increase their milk. In Europe and North America, milk weed was used to treat amoebic dysentery. An infusion of milk weed is used traditionally in East Africa as a diuretic and in West Africa, it is mostly used for high blood pressure and for swellings. More recently, especially in the Philippines, milk weed is being popularised as a treatment for dengue fever.

Modern Research and Uses

Most of the studies carried out on milk weed confirm many of the traditional uses, particularly for treating asthma and other bronchial disorders. It has been confirmed that milk weed can relax the bronchial tubes, is an expectorant and also mildly sedative.

A study carried out in Nigeria showed that a water extract of milk weed was as effective in its diuretic spectrum as acetazolamide, a commonly prescribed diuretic. In research at the UWI in Jamaica, milk weed was shown to have angiotensin-converting enzyme (ACE) inhibiting properties, which explains its effectiveness in reducing blood pressure.

Research has also confirmed that milk weed has significant anti-diabetic and cholesterol-lowering effects. The herb has also exhibited anti-microbial, anti-inflammatory and anti-tumour activity in studies on mice. Another study concluded that methanol extracts of milk weed had significant antiretroviral effects on HIV-1, HIV-2 cell lines in vitro, but aqueous extracts were less effective. Milk weed is yet another herb that needs further research to fully explore its medicinal properties.

Plant Chemicals

Plant chemicals in milk weed include: flavonoids; alkaloids; phenols; terpenoids; steroids; tannins.

Caution!

People on blood pressure medication should not use milk weed without having their pressure monitored. Some people might be allergic to the sap/latex so test a small area of skin before prolonged use on skin.

MORINGA – Moringa oleifera – Moringaceae

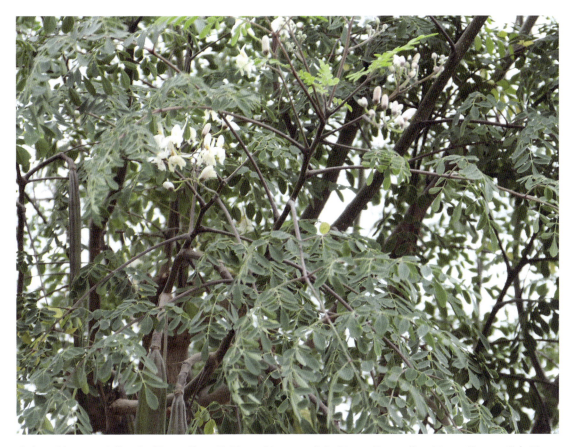

Other Names: Miracle Tree; Benoil Tree; Horseradish Tree; Benzolive Tree; Drumstick Tree; Mlonge; Muringai; Kalamungay; Moonga; Shiferaw; Rawag; Ewe-Igbale; Nebedayo

Brief Description

Moringa is native to Northern India but can now be found in a variety of geographical areas ranging from tropical islands to more arid parts of Australia and Africa. The tree grows quickly and is relatively slender with drooping branches and has pale green, feathery, compound leaves. The flowers range from creamy-white to yellow, and bear long triangular pods, which can be from 30-50 centimetres in length. The 'winged' seeds are covered with a white membrane.

Parts Used: Leaves; Flowers; Fruits; Seeds; Oil; Bark; Roots

Traditional Uses

Moringa was first introduced into Jamaica in 1784 and was grown for the oil, which was used as a lubricant for fine machinery such as watches (see below). In Jamaica, the seeds are chewed to relieve stomach problems, such as cramps and constipation, and the leaves are said to be effective in treating stomach ulcers and as a general cure-all.

Moringa has a long history of medicinal, therapeutic and cosmetic use in India, Egypt and the Far East. The bark and roots are used to treat rheumatism, venomous bites, as an antiseptic for strengthening the lungs and to restore sexual function. The leaf juice is used for viral illnesses, including colds and cold sores; to lower blood pressure and to regulate the thyroid gland.

In Ghana, a tea of young moringa leaves is drunk to relieve asthma and painful joints, and externally for boils, glandular swelling and for skin problems. Moringa leaves are also used as a poultice to relieve headaches and to dress ulcerated sores. In India, a decoction of the roots is used to prevent pregnancy, and a poultice made from pounded roots is applied to inflamed joints and swellings.

Modern Research and Uses

For more than 50 years, there have been a number of studies on the effectiveness of moringa for various health conditions. Most of these studies have looked at traditional uses of moringa for stomach ulcers, tumours and for its antibiotic and anti-fungal properties. The findings from these studies support many of traditional uses. In animal and cell-culture experiments, moringa has been reported as having anti-inflammatory, antioxidant, antiviral and anti-cancer properties.

Studies have reported that moringa extracts are effective against Staphylococcus aureus and streptococcus aureus bacteria. One of the plant compounds in moringa, pterygospermin, is thought to be responsible for its antibiotic properties, which might explain why moringa has demonstrated significant effect on H. pylori in animal studies. Moringa in all forms has also been shown to have laxative activity.

Other studies of extracts of various parts of the moringa plant provide evidence that it can help lower blood pressure, blood sugar and cholesterol levels, which can be useful in improving overall cardiovascular health. A recent study found that an alcohol extract of moringa seeds showed strong analgesic activity. Moringa is also reported to have significant effects on liver and bladder conditions, but further studies are needed to determine how these effects work.

Plant Chemicals

Plant chemicals in moringa include: alkaloids; flavonoids; phenols; steroids; pterygospermin; carotenoids; glycosides; terpenoids; cinnamates; essential oils.

Other Uses

The main use for moringa is as a highly nutritious foodstuff. Fresh raw moringa leaves contain 6.7g of protein, 1.7% fat and 13.4g of carbohydrates. Other nutrients include high levels of calcium and vitamins A, B and C. Most of the vitamins, especially C, are heat sensitive. The dried leaf powder contains more than 27g of protein, with a good balance of amino acids, 2.3% fat and 38g of carbohydrates: it also has very high levels of calcium, potassium, magnesium, iron, zinc, selenium and copper. The dried leaves are particularly rich in pro-vitamin A.

The young seed pod, which can be eaten like a vegetable, contains vitamin C, a range of B vitamins, amino acids and minerals, such as copper and potassium, and is higher in fibre than the fresh leaves. Moringa seeds can be eaten raw, but are mostly used for oil extraction, as the seeds contain, on average, 40% oil, which is sweet, non-sticking, non-drying and does not get rancid easily. Moringa oil has a high percentage of unsaturated fats (82%) in comparison to saturated fats (13%) and is rich in essential fatty acids.

In the early nineteenth century, there were calls in the Jamaican Parliament for the expansion of moringa farms. The oil was said to be good enough to use as a salad dressing but, more importantly, for lighting purposes, as it is odourless and burns with little or no smoke. The oil from moringa seeds is reported to have anti-ageing properties for the skin and can condition and strengthen the hair. It would therefore be ideal for making cosmetics, hair and skincare products.

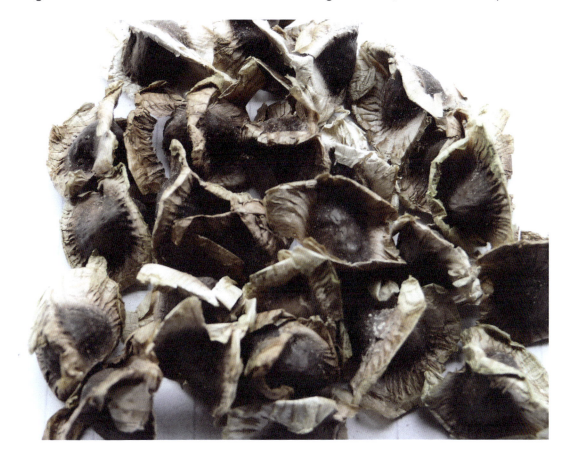

The seedcake left over from the oil extraction process can be used as a low-cost water purification medium and fertiliser. The leaf juice and leaves are also good additives to soil health. The seed powder can be used to clarify sugar cane juice and honey without heating.

Moringa leaves can also provide nutritious fodder for cattle. The timber of the moringa tree can be used in the manufacture of rayon and cellophane, and the bark produces a blue dye.

The moringa tree has the potential to provide the raw materials for a wide variety of medicinal, nutritional and commercial products. The trees grow easily in almost all parts of the island and need little input to flourish. Moringa offers the opportunity to develop value-added products for local use and export.

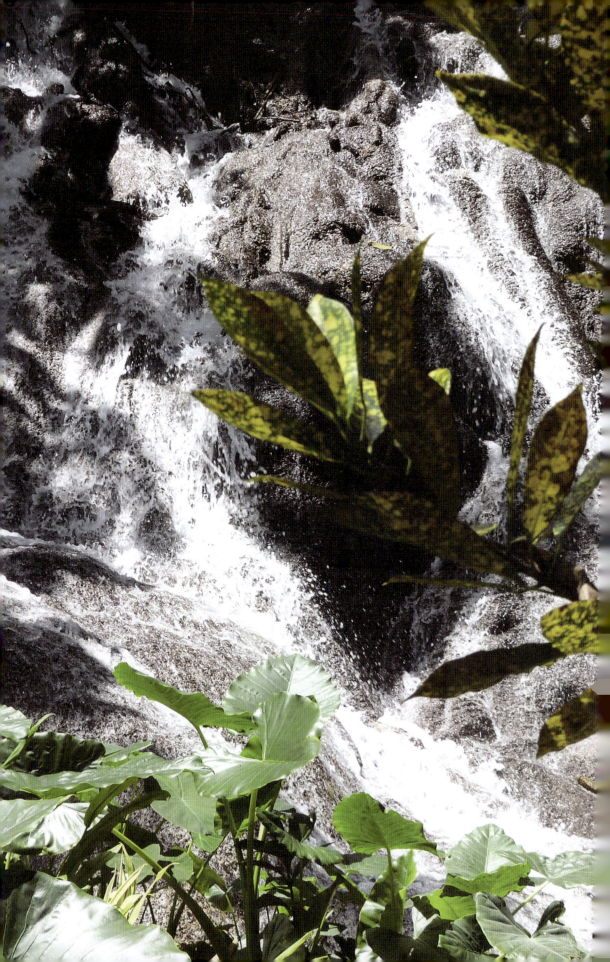

NICKEL – *Caesalpinia bonducella* – Caesalpiniaceae

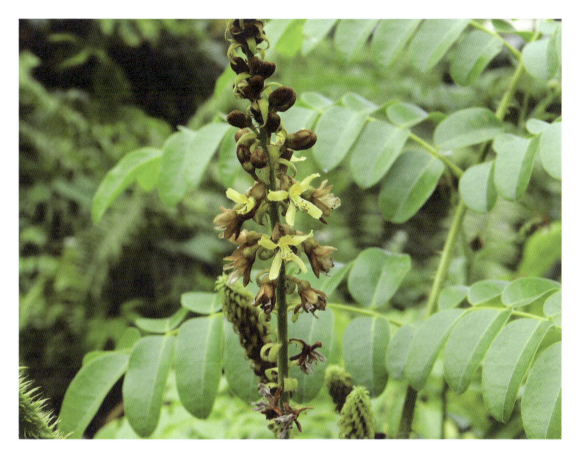

Other Names: Nicker, Nikkar Nuts, Nichor, Nichol Seeds, Oware-amba, Fever Nut; Kantkarej; Kalumbibit; Komwe; Banduc; Mate de Costa; Yeux a Chat

Brief Description

The thorny nickel bush is a creeping vine that can reach heights of up to nine metres. Nickel grows in the West Indies, Africa, India and other tropical parts of the world. The pods are covered with prickles and contain hard shiny yellow or grey seeds around the size of a marble.

Parts Used: Seeds, Roots, Stems

Traditional Uses

In Jamaica, nickel is traditionally dried, ground and brewed like coffee. This is reputed to be effective in treating diabetes, high blood pressure and kidney problems. Nickel is also said to be good for gonorrhoea and fever. The grey seed is thought to be more effective than the yellow one for healing.

The seed or nut is used in India to treat fevers, as an aphrodisiac and to prevent the return of recurrent fevers, such as malaria. They also use a decoction of the leaves internally for gastric disorders including colitis. In the Philippines, an ointment made from the seeds mixed with castor oil is applied to swellings and for arthritis. A decoction of the roasted seeds is thought to be good for asthma and other respiratory conditions. In Ghana, nickel is best known as an aphrodisiac and treatment for sterility. The pounded roots and stems are soaked in palm wine for these purposes. The seed powder is applied to ulcers and when applied to the eyes is said to prevent spots forming on the cornea.

Modern Research and Uses

Some studies have been carried out on nickel and they have confirmed many of its traditional uses, especially for diabetes. One study carried out in India showed that a nickel extract was particularly effective in reducing blood sugar levels in rats with diabetes. Nickel's hypoglycaemic effects were observed in other studies with animals as well as in laboratory tests.

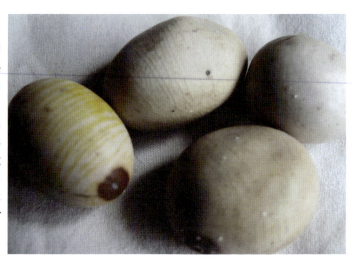

Other studies have reported significant anti-tumour and antioxidant activity in tests on mice and in vitro experiments. Nickel is also said to be diuretic, anti-periodic and anthelmintic. Research on animal models has demonstrated that both an ethanol extract of the seed and the nickel seed oil have significant effectiveness in reducing fever and relieving pain.

The traditional use of nickel for malaria has been supported by a recent study in which the aqueous ethanol extract of the plants roots was found to be effective in treating malaria in mice. This finding offers hopes of identifying new compounds which can be developed to combat malaria, particularly in developing countries where nickel grows abundantly.

Findings from one study showed that nickel has immuno-modulating activity. Researchers at UWI in Jamaica isolated a furanoditerpene, called caesalpine F, but it has not been tested in terms of its bio-activity.

Plant Chemicals

Plant chemicals in nickel include: alkaloids; tannins; saponins; steroids; glucosides; terpenoids; flavonoids; glycosides.

Other Uses

Nickel yields an oil that has not yet been exploited for its potential commercial uses. The nickel seeds are the original seeds used to play the African game Oware.

Caution!

People with diabetes should not take nickel without having their blood sugar levels monitored.

NONI – Morinda citrifolia – Rubiaceae

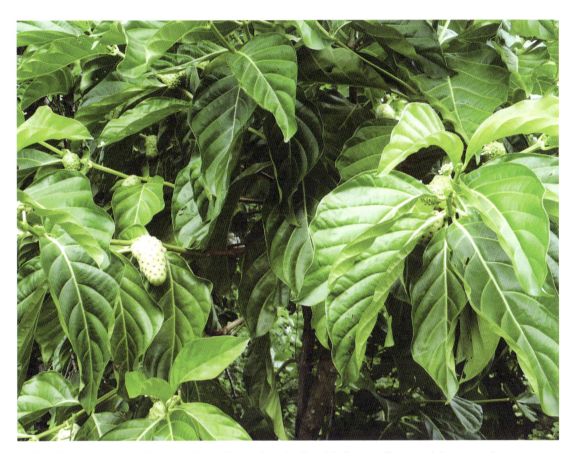

Other Names: Duppy Soursop; Dog Dumpling; Indian Mulberry; Pomme Macaque; Apatot

Brief Description

Noni is a small tree or shrub, originating in Polynesia that can grow up to eight metres in height with leaves of up to 35 centimetres long. It has whitish flowers which bear a fruit that looks like a small, green, oval breadfruit and can be up to 15 centimetres long. When mature, the fruits become whitish and almost translucent with a distinctive, unpleasant smell.

Parts Used: Leaves; Fruits; Bark; Roots

Traditional Uses

In Jamaica the fruit of the noni was not traditionally used for healing. The leaves are used as a poultice for headaches, wounds, and to relieve joint pains. Similar use was made of the leaves in other Caribbean islands. The bark and roots were also used in Jamaica as an ingredient in popular roots tonics. In recent years, the fermented fruit juice has been marketed as a cure-all.

The noni plant, including the leaves and fruits, is used traditionally in Polynesia to treat a variety of health conditions, from cancer to lesser infections, and to aid in recovery from illness. The leaves and leaf juice, applied topically are thought to be effective in treating chronic skin ulcers, gout and snake bites. Taken internally, the leaf juice or infusion is used mainly for dysentery, hypertension and tuberculosis.

In India and parts of Southeast Asia, noni leaves and fruits are used internally for fever, constipation and liver problems and externally for wounds, abscesses, arthritis, swellings and gout. In Africa, a tea made from noni leaves and sometimes combined with the bark is used for malaria, fever and pain.

Modern Research and Uses

The juice from the fruit has, in recent years, been promoted in the West as a cure-all for everything from depression to cancer, and this has made some people sceptical about its health benefits. Various studies carried out in different parts of the world have confirmed many of the traditional uses of what is referred to as Tahitian Noni Juice ®, or TNJ.

A review carried out by Wang in 2002 reported that TNJ has significant analgesic, anti-inflammatory, and immune-boosting properties. It was also confirmed that there is strong evidence that TNJ enhanced the effects of cancer drugs and improved the overall health and well-being of people who have degenerative diseases. Other studies have shown that extracts of noni leaves and fermented noni juice can reduce blood sugar levels, protect the liver and may prevent or delay the development of cancer. There is however little evidence at present to suggest that noni can treat cancers.

Noni has been shown to be beneficial in boosting the immune system, reducing inflammation and repairing and regenerating cells. Noni has the potential to contribute to treating cases of arthritis and other inflammatory conditions; heart and circulatory problems. In animal experiments, ethanol extracts of the roots and the fruit were reported to be analgesic, antibiotic and antiviral. In an in vitro study carried out in the Philippines, noni leaf extracts were very effective against the mycobacterium that causes tuberculosis and was just marginally less effective than one of the leading TB drugs.

Noni leaves are also reported to be useful in treating intestinal parasites and are rich in a number of vitamins, minerals and plant chemicals which can maintain and improve overall health. Hopefully, research will continue into the many active plant chemicals in noni.

Plant Chemicals

Plant chemicals in noni include: alkaloids; steroids; phenols; carotenoids; sulphides; glycosides; saponins; glucosides; coumarins; allantoin.

Caution!

No significant side effects have been reported for noni, but it is preferable to drink the juice on an empty stomach. There are some concerns that excessive consumption of fermented noni juice may adversely affect the liver: hence the need for further research to get more

information to help people to make best use of this amazing plant.

OIL NUT – *Ricinus communis* – Euphorbiaceae

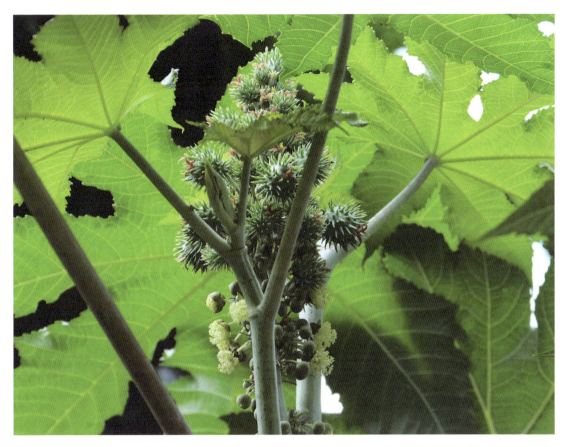

Other Names: Castor Oil; Pomaskwiti; Palma Christi; Cawapate; Huile de Ricin; Tangan-tangan; Arand; Mbalika

Brief Description

Oil nut is an evergreen shrub or small tree growing up to eight metres in height, with palm-shaped leaves up to 30 centimetres wide. The plant bears greenish flowers, which produce prickly, round pods that contain the seeds.

Parts Used: Leaves; Seeds; Roots; Oil

Traditional Uses

In Jamaica, oil nut leaves are applied externally for relief from headaches. Castor oil, which is extracted from the dried seeds of the plant, has many applications. It is used as a purgative, for skin problems and for hair and scalp problems. The oil is also used topically for sprains, bruises and inflammation.

In the Eastern Caribbean, oil nut leaves are heated and used as a poultice for the relief of inflammation, internal swelling and pain. A tea made with oil nut leaves and other herbs is used there to treat gonorrhoea. In India, oil nut leaves are used for swellings, sores and carbuncles. The oil is used as a purgative and for internal inflammations and externally for swollen breasts, dermatitis and eye problems. In parts of Africa, pounded leaves are applied to guinea worm sores to help extract the worms and a dressing made from the bark is used for wounds and hard-to-heal sores.

The seeds of the oil nut plant are used by women in parts of Nigeria, India, Pakistan and Saudi Arabia as a form of contraception. Two to five seeds are swallowed on the first day of menstruation and this is believed to prevent conception for a few months.

Modern Research and Uses

A lot of research has been carried out on the toxicity of ricin, the main active plant chemical in oil nut, which can be deadly if ingested. Ricin-derived immuno-toxins (RDIs) have been used in bone marrow transplant procedures, to reduce the likelihood of rejection of bone marrow in host patients. These procedures have proven successful in some cases where steroids have failed. There have been studies to look at the potential of RDIs to target cancer cells, but clinical trials have been less successful, due mainly to leaking blood vessels, which result from the procedure. Research is, however, continuing in the use of RDIs in treating cancers and AIDS.

Oil nut leaf and root extracts have shown analgesic effects, confirming their traditional use to relieve headaches. In other studies, ethanol extracts of oil nut roots, leaves and stems demonstrated anti-inflammatory, antioxidant, anti-asthmatic and hepato-protective properties. The root extracts were also effective in reducing blood sugar levels, but only in large doses. In vitro tests showed that methanol extracts of oil nut leaves were more effective against bacteria than aqueous or ethanol extracts. However, both methanol and aqueous extracts proved to be anti-fungal.

A number of studies have been carried out which have confirmed the ability of oil nut seed extracts to prevent conception in female rats and rabbits. Research has also indicated that extracts from both the roots and seeds of the oil nut reduced the sperm count in male rats. These findings suggest that further research is needed to identify the mechanisms and plant chemicals that are involved, which could lead to the development of viable contraceptives from the oil nut plant.

Plant Chemicals

Plant chemicals in oil nut include: ricin; flavonoids; steroids; saponins; glycosides; terpenoids; alkaloids; glucosides; tannins; squalene.

Other Uses

One of the main reasons that castor oil is so widely used, is the fact that it does not congeal at low temperatures. Castor oil is used to make soaps, various cosmetics, candles, crayons, varnishes, lubricating oils, high-performance fuels, polyamide fibre and leather preservative.

The oil has long been used as fuel for lighting and has huge potential as a bio fuel. Residue from the oil extraction process is used in the manufacture of fertilisers, caulking for treating timber and to prevent termite infestation. Apart from the plant's commercial uses, latest research suggests that oil nut trees could play a crucial role in the absorption of carbon dioxide in the atmosphere, reducing the levels of this greenhouse gas.

More recently Ricinus communis polyurethane (RCP) has been developed for use in surgical procedures, where biocompatible material to repair or reconstruct bone or tissue is required. Studies so far suggest that RCP is a viable and sustainable alternative to demineralised bone and titanium implants.

Oil nut trees grow easily across Jamaica in even the poorest soil and need neither fertilisers nor insecticides. This plant offers a wide range of opportunities for the development of products for both local use and export.

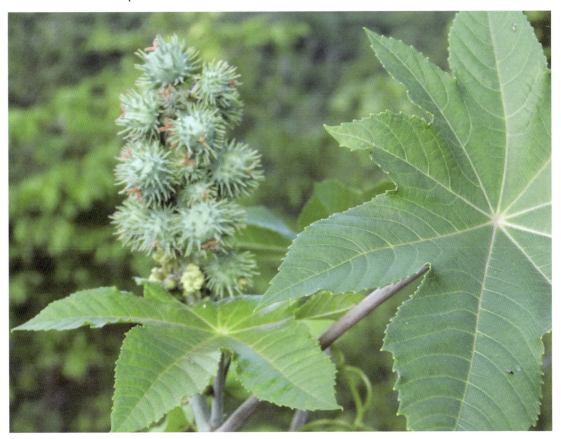

Caution!

The main plant chemical in oil nut is ricin, which is very poisonous. Ricin is not transferred into the oil made from the seeds. Research has indicated that one milligram of ricin can kill an adult and that just one seed can kill a child. If the seed of the castor plant is swallowed and the seed coat is not damaged, it can pass through the body without danger. However if the seed is damaged or chewed, ricin will be absorbed into the intestines, which can lead to severe poisoning and death. Ricin is regarded as a hazardous substance and is banned in many countries.

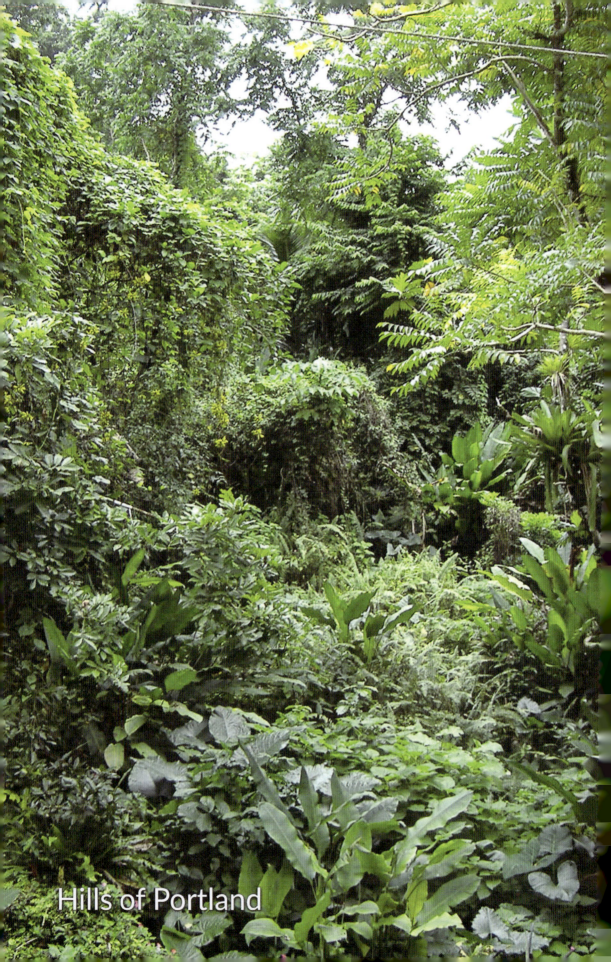

Hills of Portland

PASSION FRUIT – *Passiflora edulis* – *Passifloraceae*

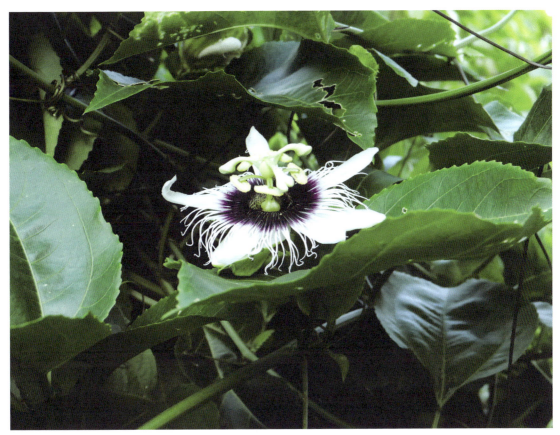

Other Names: Passion Flower; Maracuja; Granadilla; Love-in-a-mist; Maypop; Parcha; Sweet Cup; Pasyonarya

Brief Description

Passion fruit is native to Brazil but is now grown in many tropical and subtropical parts of the world. There are many varieties of passion fruit including hybrids. The plant is a woody, climbing vine that spreads over its host tree. The vine has three-lobed leaves and bears beautiful, fragrant white to purple flowers. The passion fruit is green and egg shaped, varying in size and most varieties turn yellow or purple and wrinkle slightly when ripe.

Parts Used: Leaves; Whole Plant; Fruits; Rind

Traditional Uses

The passion fruit plant has been in recorded use for over 400 years, since it was introduced into Europe. It was used traditionally in the Amazon for pain relief, insomnia and as a sedative. Passiflora, as it was commonly called, has been used popularly for sleep and anxiety disorders for a few centuries.

In Jamaica, both the leaves and vine are used for colds and for kidney problems. In the Eastern Caribbean, passion fruit is used for sore throats and kidney troubles. In South America, passion fruit has long been prized for its calming, sedative effects. It is used there to treat many conditions, such as tension headaches, nerve pain, muscle spasms, insomnia, menstrual problems and as a nerve tonic. In some countries in Central America, passion fruit is regarded as an aphrodisiac and also used for lowering blood pressure.

Modern Research and Uses

Research on passion fruit plant has been going on for more than 100 years, and many of the traditional uses of this herb have been validated. Passion fruit's tranquilising, sedative and pain-relieving properties have been clinically documented since the early twentieth century. Other studies have concluded that passion fruit plant has anti-spasmodic, hypotensive, anti-inflammatory, anti-anxiety and diuretic effects.

In Europe and North America, there are herbal medicines with 'passiflora' in them, mainly for sleep problems, nervous exhaustion and to lower blood pressure. Passion fruit leaves are also reported to be effective in treating irritable bowel syndrome, pre-menstrual tension and tachycardia. This is most likely due to its anti-spasmodic and sedative properties.

Passion fruit plant is also useful for menopausal symptoms and convulsions. Ethanol extracts of the leaves exhibited high antioxidant activity in lab tests. In South America, passion fruit juice is currently used to relieve symptoms of hyperactivity in children, for asthma, coughs and other bronchial problems.

One study in vitro has confirmed passion fruit's potential for lowering blood pressure, by highlighting the angiotensin-converting enzyme (ACE) inhibiting properties of extracts from both the leaves and fruits.

Recent studies on the rind of the passion fruit on rats have shown that the powdered rind extract lowered blood sugar, blood pressure, cholesterol and helped in weight reduction. The rind is rich in soluble fibres, such as pectins and mucilage, which play a key role in digestive processes.

Plant Chemicals

Plant chemicals in passion fruit plant include: alkaloids; flavonoids; glycosides; phenols; glucosides; glycosides; terpenoids; steroids; coumarins.

Other Uses

The passion fruit itself is widely used to make drinks, preserves and confectionery and the fruit is grown on a commercial scale to make these products. The fruit and its derivatives are a rich source of niacin, riboflavin and potassium. The seeds produce an oil that is similar to soya or sunflower oils. It is a good emollient, rich in vitamins C and E, linoleic and oleic acids. This oil has the potential for use in the food, pharmaceutical and cosmetic industries.

> **Caution!**
>
> Due to the passion fruit plant's reported hypotensive activity, it is important to have your blood pressure monitored by a health professional, and caution should be exercised if using prescribed medication.

PEPPER ELDER – *Piper amalago* – *Piperaceae*

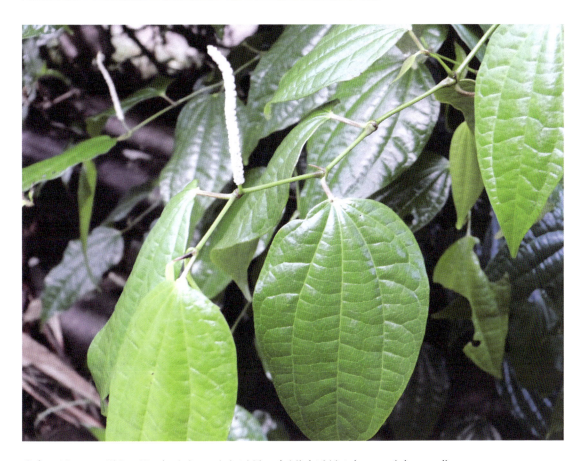

Other Names: Shine Bush; Jointy; Joint Wood; Night Watchman; Jaborandi-manso

Brief Description

Pepper elder is a small tree or shrub, growing up to three metres in height, with woody, knotty stems. The leaves are dark green, veined, shiny and can be up to 15 centimetres in length. The tiny berries bear on erect stalks.

Parts Used: Leaves; Berries; Stems

Traditional Uses

In Jamaica, pepper elder is traditionally used to treat nausea and vomiting, and boiled with ginger for stomach ache. It is also used for colds, flu, fever and pain, including painful menstruation. The leaves and twigs can be boiled and drunk as a tea or used as a bath for these conditions. Pepper elder was also thought to be a stimulant, hence the name 'night watchman'. The leaves and stems of pepper elder are also considered to be beneficial for flatulence and as a blood tonic. In the Eastern Caribbean, pepper elder is used to treat colds, flu and for a variety of stomach disorders.

Pepper elder is used in folk medicine in Central and South America for joint pains, swellings, to relieve pain and for stomach problems. In Brazil, it is also used traditionally as a diuretic and for preventing and treating kidney stones.

Modern Research and Uses

Relatively little research has been carried out on pepper elder. In an early study in 1962, in Jamaica, it was reported that pepper elder can be useful in the treatment of high blood pressure. A more recent study in Brazil has concluded that an ethanolic extract from pepper elder significantly increased urine output and also inhibited formation of calcium oxalate deposits, which can lead to the formation of kidney stones.

Recent research has also confirmed that pepper elder has anti-inflammatory properties in topical application that is as effective as indomethacin, a non-steroidal anti-inflammatory drug (NSAID). Another study of pepper elder has reported that it has plant chemicals that could be useful in the treatment of cancer, but these findings are at an early stage, requiring further research.

Essential oil can be extracted from the leaf, stem, root and berries of the pepper elder and one study in Brazil found that the essential oil contained more than 50 compounds. The essential oil exhibited anti-fungal activity on a number of Candida strains as well as anti-microbial and antioxidant effects. In animal experiments in Guatemala, extracts of pepper elder leaves demonstrated anti-anxiety effects, which suggest that the traditional use of this plant to treat anxiety-related disorders may have some pharmacological basis.

Plant Chemicals

Plant chemicals in pepper elder include: alkaloids; terpenoids; flavonoids; steroids; lignans; essential oils.

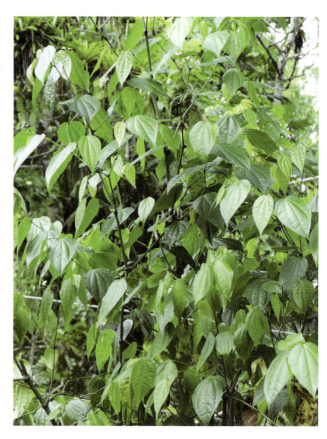

Other Uses

Pepper elder leaves and berries are used as a spice, especially among the Maroons in Portland, Jamaica, who use it to jerk pork. The berries can be used as a substitute for black pepper.

Pepper elder oil and key compounds in the plant extracts have been confirmed in research as having insecticidal effects on insects and on the larvae of the Aedes aegyptii mosquito, which can transmit dengue fever, chikungunya, Zika virus and yellow fever.

Pepper elder was traditionally used to preserve dead bodies in rural areas of Jamaica, prior to refrigeration.

Caution!

People on blood pressure medication should not use pepper elder unless under the supervision of a healthcare professional.

PIMENTO – *Pimenta dioica* – Myrataceae

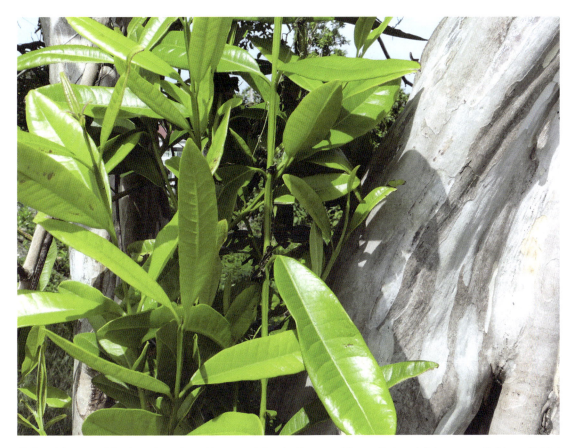

Other Names: Allspice; Jamaican Pepper; Myrtle Pepper; Toute Epice; Malagueta; Bakhar; Fulful Ifranji

Brief Description

Pimento is native to the West Indies, mainly Jamaica and Cuba, but now grows in many tropical parts of the world. The tree can reach up to ten metres in height and has an unusual whitish bark, with shiny green, oval leaves, similar to the guava tree. The tree flowers from June to August, and the berries these produce are harvested and dried before they ripen. Pimento got the name 'allspice' because of its smell, which is a mixture of nutmeg, cinnamon and clove.

Parts Used: Leaves; Berries (ripe and unripe dried); Oil

Traditional Uses

Jamaica is renowned for producing the best quality pimento and both the ripe and dried pimento berries are used there in traditional healing. The ripe and unripe berries are soaked in rum with ginger and used both internally and externally to relieve pains, including stomach ache, toothache and menstrual pains. A tea made from the leaves is said to be good for the blood.

On other Caribbean islands such as Cuba, Haiti and the Dominican Republic, pimento is used by itself or in combination with other herbs for a wide range of health problems including:

diabetes, nausea, gastro-intestinal ailments, depression, muscle and joint pains, anxiety and sinus infections. Both the berries and leaves are used to make a tea, and the ground seed powder is made into a paste and applied externally as a poultice for painful joints and muscles.

Modern Research and Uses

Pimento is still used today in much the same way it has been used traditionally. Identification of the active plant chemicals confirm that pimento is aromatic and carminative and is useful in the treatment of gastro-intestinal problems, such as diarrhoea and flatulence and as an aid to digestion. The essential oil made from pimento has been proven to be effective in cases of stress, depression, and nervous exhaustion.

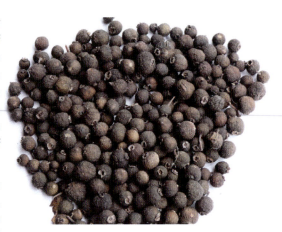

Eugenol, one of the main plant chemicals in both the berries and the oil, has local anaesthetic, analgesic and antiseptic properties. Pimento can stop chills, improve circulation, and is useful for colds, flu and for menstrual pains. Pimento oil, which can be extracted from both the unripe berries and the leaves, is used in similar ways to clove oil to treat toothaches, rheumatism and muscular pains and is antioxidant. One study has indicated that one plant chemical in the leaves of the pimento, peduncalagin, has anti-tumour and antioxidant effects. Pimento leaves also have antibacterial, anti-fungal and hypotensive properties. Findings from research have confirmed most of the traditional and current uses of pimento in all forms.

New compounds have been identified in pimento berries, and one in particular, ericifolin, has been found to have significant effects on prostate and breast cancer cells, in both in vitro and in vivo experiments.

Plant Chemicals

Plant chemicals in pimento include: phenols; terpenoids; glycosides; flavonoids; glucosides; phenylpropanoids; essential oils.

Other Uses

Pimento is mainly used as spice and was particularly important pre-refrigeration, when it was a key ingredient in preparations to preserve meats and vegetables. Pimento is still widely used in the food industry where it adds flavour to well-known sauces and condiments, in particular jerk seasoning, which is now internationally renowned. A liqueur from the ripe berries is still made in Jamaica. Due to the aromatic and therapeutic oil in pimento, it is widely used in perfumes and cosmetic products.

Pimento oil has been reported as being very effective in killing cow ticks and also in eradicating nematodes.

Caution!

Pimento oil should not be taken internally without professional supervision. Care should also be exercised when using pimento oil externally, even when diluted, as some people are sensitive to plant chemicals in the oil, especially eugenol.

QUEEN'S FLOWER – Lagerstroemia speciosa – Lythraceae

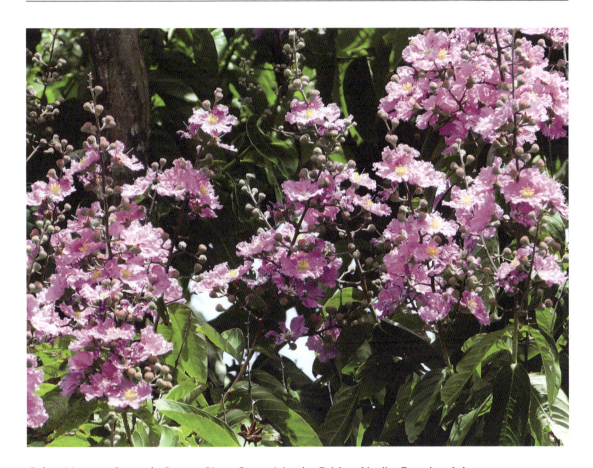

Other Names: Queen's Crape; Giant Crape Myrtle; Pride of India; Banaba; Arjuna

Brief Description

Queen's flower is a deciduous tropical flowering tree that is native to southern Asia, which now grows in the Philippines, Southeast Asia and India. The tree is cultivated widely in tropical parts of the world for shade and as an ornamental and can grow up to 20 metres tall. Queen's flower has coarse oblong leaves that can be 15 to 25 centimetres long; the tree bears beautiful bunches of pink, purple or purplish-pink flowers. The fruits are small, oval and split when mature.

Parts Used: Leaves; Fruits; Flowers; Bark

Traditional Uses

Queen's flower is not used traditionally in Jamaican herbal medicine, but the tree is grown there, so it is useful to know about its medicinal value. In the Philippines, the dried leaves and fruits of the queen's flower, known there as banaba, are widely used to treat diabetes and aid weight loss. In Japan, it is referred to as 'slimming tea', and in other parts of the Far East, the flowers and leaves of the plant are used to treat constipation and a decoction of the leaves for urinary and kidney problems. The bark decoction is traditionally used to treat diarrhoea and is also reputed to be effective in cases of fever.

Modern Research and Uses

Research on queen's flower was first carried out in 1940 to assess its traditional use for diabetes, but it was not until the 1990s that international interest in the plant really grew. In several animal studies, both water- and alcohol-based extracts of the leaves and fruits of queen's flower tree were effective in reducing blood sugar levels. Extracts from the leaves have also been used for weight loss and to reduce cholesterol levels. Corosolic acid, one of the key plant chemicals in queen's flower, has anti-inflammatory, antiviral, antioxidant as well as hypoglycaemic properties.

Studies have confirmed traditional uses of the plant, but scientists have recently tried to identify which plant chemicals in the queen's flower are responsible for these effects. Some researchers thought that the triterpenoid, corosolic acid, was the key compound in the plant. However, more recent research has highlighted the significant activity of a compound in the tannic acid, which is present in the leaves, especially the older ones, and in the fruits. This plant chemical called penta-O-galloyl-D-glucopyranose (PGG) also has anti-cancer, anti-inflammatory, antiviral and antioxidant properties. Another plant chemical in queen's flower, valoneic acid dilactone (VAD), has proved to be effective in treating gout by lowering uric acid levels. A tea of the leaves is also useful as a diuretic and mild purgative.

Plant Chemicals

The plant chemicals in queen's flower include: tannins; flavonoids; terpenoids; coumarin; steroids; lignans.

Other Uses

Queen's flower tree is usually planted for shade and for the showy flowers. When mature, the tree provides good quality timber which can be used to make furniture, boats and in house building.

Caution!

For people who are already on medication for diabetes, queen's flower should only be used under professional supervision to avoid sudden and significant reduction in blood sugar levels, which can lead to a diabetic coma.

RAMGOAT REGULAR – Turnera ulmifolia – Turneraceae

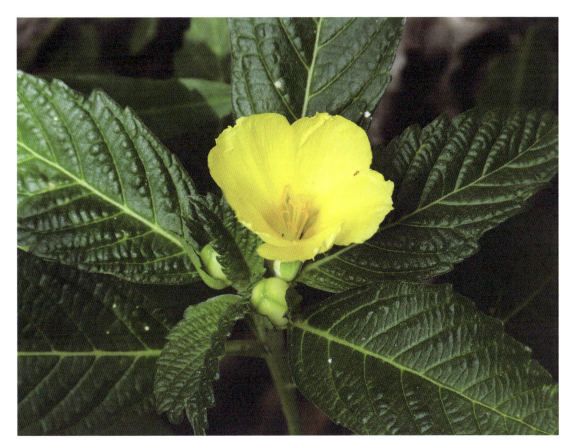

Other Names: Ramgoat Dashalong; Holly Rose; Chanana; Cuban Buttercup; Yellow Alder

Brief Description

Ramgoat regular is native to Central America and the Caribbean but now grows in Africa and Asia. The shrub can grow up to 1.5 metres in height and has bright green leaves and yellow flowers. Ramgoat regular is related to damiana, which is similar in appearance and shares some of its medicinal properties.

Parts Used: Leaves; Flowers; Whole Plant

Traditional Uses

In Jamaica, ramgoat regular is a traditional remedy for colds. The tea is also used as a general tonic for debility, constipation, fevers and externally for prickly heat. Ramgoat regular is reputed to cause abortions, so care must be exercised when using it. Some people regard this herb as an enhancer of male performance, hence the common name. This might be due to the similarities between ramgoat regular and damiana which is renowned as an aphrodisiac.

In the Eastern Caribbean, ramgoat regular is boiled and taken for gastro-intestinal problems, including diarrhoea, piles and menstrual cramps. It is also mixed with carry mi seed and used for fevers, colds and for expulsion of the afterbirth. In Brazil, tea made from ramgoat regular is traditionally used to treat gastric problems, including gastric and duodenal ulcers and as an anti-inflammatory agent. The flowers are also used in some South and Central America countries to treat wounds. In parts of Asia, ramgoat regular is traditionally used for digestive disorders, liver problems and diabetes.

Modern Research and Uses

Recent research in Brazil has confirmed the traditional use of ramgoat regular for both duodenal and gastric ulcers. Phenolic compounds in the herb are thought to be responsible for these anti-ulcerogenic properties.

Another study in Brazil reported that ramgoat regular has significant antioxidant and anti-inflammatory properties. These properties might explain why ramgoat regular is reputed to be effective in treating degenerative diseases such as rheumatoid arthritis and other musculoskeletal conditions.

Antibacterial activity has been identified in laboratory tests against a number of bacteria, including salmonella and E. coli. A study on rats in India found that a methanol extract of ramgoat regular had significant hypoglycaemic effects, which confirms one of the traditional uses of the herb. Further tests are recommended to find out which compounds are responsible for these effects.

Plant Chemicals

Plant chemicals in ramgoat regular include: phenols; alkaloids; flavonoids; glycosides; steroids; glucosides; terpenoids; essential oils.

Caution!

Ramgoat regular should not to be used in pregnancy due to its reputation as an abortifacient.

SAGE – *Lantana camara* – Verbenaceae

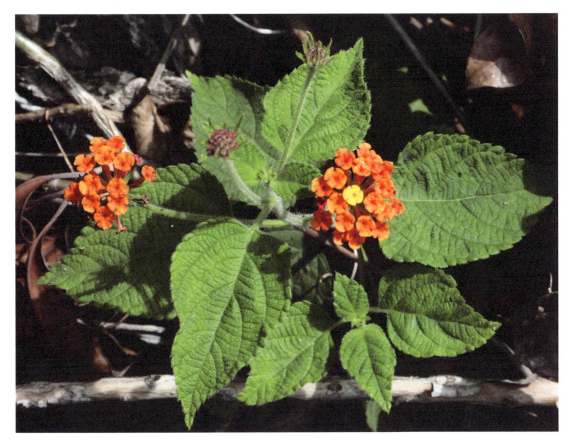

Other Names: White Sage; Wild Sage; Kayakit; Sauge; Ma Bizou; Ma-ying Tan; Kantutay; Tickberry; Spanish Flag; Umphema; Tea Plant; Mutukululu; Coronitas

Brief Description

Sage is a spreading shrub that can grow up to two metres in height. The small leaves have a rough surface and the plant bears beautiful clusters of flowers. According to the variety, these can range from red, orange and yellow to purple pink and cream. Sage bears small green berries which turn black when ripe. The plant is very aromatic.

Parts Used: Leaves; Stems; Roots; Oil; Flowers

Traditional Uses

Sage is used traditionally in Jamaica as a remedy for colds and fever. It is also used to relieve morning sickness and painful periods. Sage was also reputed to be effective in treating gonorrhoea, measles, chicken pox and sores. In the Eastern Caribbean, a juice of the sage leaf is used to treat dysentery and jaundice. The leaves are usually boiled and used as a bath for measles and chicken pox to relieve itching.

Sage is widely used around the world, and most parts of the plant have medicinal properties. In Africa and India the root is used to treat malaria, chikungunya, dengue and rheumatism, and the stem is boiled and applied to skin rashes. A decoction of the leaves is considered effective for colds, coughs, asthma and fever and the oil used as an insecticide and insect repellent. Sage is used for a wide range of health problems in Ghana and is very valued as a healing herb, especially to treat bronchitis, diarrhoea and skin ulcers.

In Indonesia the leaves are pounded and used as a poultice to reduce swellings and treat wounds. In the Philippines, a decoction of the leaves and roots is favoured for treating toothaches and asthma. The leaf oil is applied topically to relieve rheumatism and for skin conditions, such as eczema and dermatitis. Wherever sage grows, it is used for similar conditions and is valued as a healing herb.

Modern Research and Uses

Over recent years, there have been many studies carried out on different parts of the sage plant. Some have shown that sage has anti-tetanus, hypotensive, anti-microbial, antiseptic, anti-spasmodic, cytotoxic and anti-tumour properties. A study in India confirmed that a sage leaf extract demonstrated significant anti-tumour effects on a range of cancer cells in laboratory tests. Sage also has antibacterial effects and research undertaken at the UWI reported that sage extracts were effective against Staphylococcus aureus, Staphylococcus epidermis and streptococcus A, B and D.

One study in Uganda showed that a methanol extract of sage leaves had significant activity against a resistant strain of tuberculosis. Sage has also recently been reported to be effective against Helicobacter pylori, which is one of the main causes of stomach ulcers and also reduced the development of duodenal ulcers in rats.

Sage's traditional use as an anti-malarial has been supported by research carried out in Nigeria on mice, which showed that an ethanol extract of sage leaves had comparable effects on clearing malaria-causing parasites to the standard drug chloroquine. In another study, a sage leaf extract significantly inhibited castor-oil-induced diarrhoea in mice.

Sage oil has demonstrated high levels of antibacterial activity that could have widespread applications. Other studies have reported that sage has strong anti-inflammatory, analgesic and anti-pyretic activity. This widely available herb has many medicinal properties, and further research could lead to the development of pharmaceutical products from it.

Plant Chemicals

Plant chemicals in sage include: alkaloids; terpenoids; phenols; steroids; flavonoids; saponins; tannins; glycosides.

Other Uses

Sage grows wild in Jamaica and has good potential for the commercial production of essential oil. There is also the added opportunity of developing body care and healing products using the extracted oil. Sage is also said to be rich in potassium and phosphorous and could be used in agricultural production as green mulch.

Sage's insecticidal properties could also be an added bonus for the population at large as it can inhibit vector-borne diseases, by reducing larvicidal activity. Sage has also shown promise as an environmental preventative in the fight against the spread of malaria. In trials in Tanzania, sage planted around houses reduced the number of mosquitos inside the houses by more than 50%. This strategy could be useful in many countries where this plant grows easily and where mosquito-borne diseases, such as malaria, dengue and chikungunya, yellow fever and Zika virus are common.

SHAMY DARLING – Mimosa pudica – (Mimosaceae)

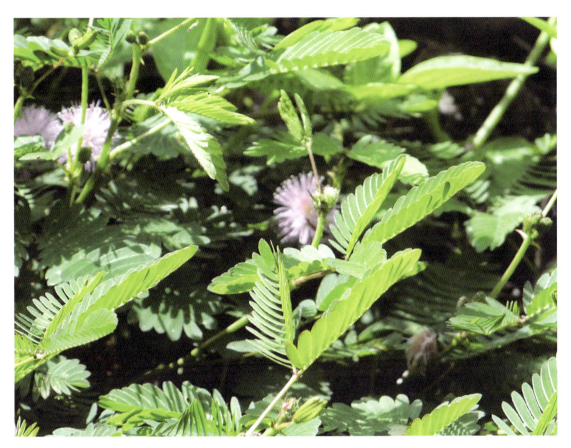

Other Names: Shamo'lady; Sensitive Plant; Kwedi; Sleeping Grass; Adormidera; Lajalu; Honteuse Femelle; Makahiya; Puteri Malu; Kpakorukwu

Brief Description

Shamy darling is native to tropical South America but now grows in many tropical regions. The plant is woody with spreading branches and has small compound leaves, which close when touched, hence the name. The stems have prickles and the plant bears small purplish flowers.

Parts Used: Leaves; Stems; Roots

Traditional Uses

Shamy darling has a long history of medicinal use in most of the countries where it grows. The leaves and roots of shamy darling are used in Jamaica to treat colds, chest and stomach pains, and as a sedative. It is traditionally combined with devil's horsewhip and strong back for colds, gonorrhoea and sexually transmitted infections. Shamy darling's stems and roots are used in the Eastern Caribbean as a purgative, emetic, and for whooping cough.

In Central American countries, shamy darling is traditionally used as a sedative and for depression. However, the Garfuna people in Guatemala use it to treat urinary infections, and in Panama, the roots and stems are beaten and boiled and used as a poultice to relieve arthritis. In Vietnamese traditional medicine, shamy darling is considered a hypnotic tranquiliser, and in India, the herb is used in treating epilepsy, as an aphrodisiac and as an anti-fertility aid. It is also commonly used on the Indian sub-continent to treat haemorrhoids and for snake bites.

In Polynesia, shamy darling is used to treat stress-related conditions and as a mild sedative. Similar use is made of the plant in Chinese herbal medicine as well as for bronchitis and asthma. The whole plant can be used as a diuretic and as a wash to treat dermatitis. In Africa, a leaf decoction is drunk for dysentery, as a tonic and applied topically for guinea worm.

Modern Research and Uses

Research on shamy darling has confirmed some of the traditional uses of the herb. In scientific trials, shamy darling extracts were found to be moderately diuretic and demonstrated an ability to promote the regeneration of nerves. A recent study has reported that shamy darling demonstrated antidepressant activity in humans.

Shamy darling is reported to be antibiotic, anti-microbial, anti-neurasthenic, anti-spasmodic, nervine, and sedative and the root extracts are said to be a strong emetic. A decoction of shamy darling has also exhibited anti-convulsant properties. Another study in mice has given some scientific basis to the traditional use of shamy darling as an anti-fertility agent. Results from the experiment showed significant reduction in the fertility of female mice which had been given a shamy darling root extract for 21 days.

Shamy darling was also used in a small-scale trial with nine female patients who had abnormal uterine bleeding. A root extract was given to them for a number of cycles and in all cases there was a marked decrease in bleeding and associated symptoms. Although further trials were planned, there are no reports of these. The initial results give credibility to the traditional use of shamy darling leaves and roots to reduce bleeding in a number of ailments.

Another traditional use of shamy darling to treat snake bites and other venom has been validated by a number of studies going back more than 30 years, which have looked at the effectiveness of the plant in neutralising various types of venom. Using both in vivo and in vitro models, different parts of the shamy darling plant have repeatedly demonstrated antivenin properties.

Plant Chemicals

Plant chemicals in shamy darling include: alkaloids; glycosides; steroids; terpenoids; tannins; flavonoids; phenols; saponins.

Other Uses

In 2011, a Nigerian researcher developed solar cells using materials which had been treated with an extract from shamy darling. The discovery offers exciting possibilities for commercial manufacturing of solar panels and other products using extracts from this widely available plant, particularly in developing countries.

> **Caution!**
>
> There have been reports that shamy darling can be toxic, if used internally for a long time or if a large amount of the herb is ingested. It is advisable to seek professional advice before using this herb for an extended period. Avoid use if pregnant or trying to get pregnant.

SOUR SOP – *Annona muricata* – Annonaceae

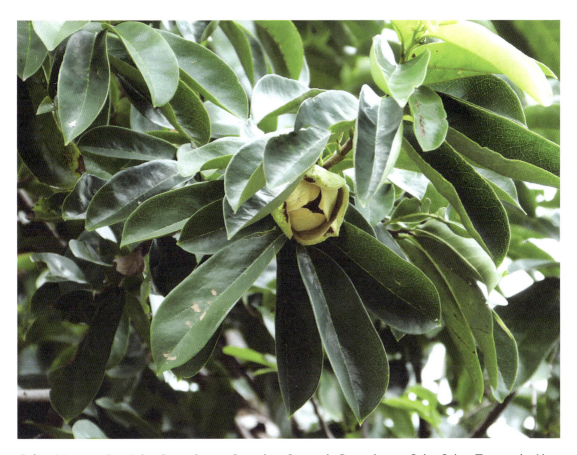

Other Names: Graviola; Guanabana; Catoche; Corosol; Guayabano; Saba Saba; Zuurzack; Abo; Apre

Brief Description

Sour sop is native to South America but is now grown throughout the Caribbean, Central America, Southeast Asia and the Pacific region. The tree grows up to eight metres in height with shiny, oblong, leaves, which can be from 10-20 centimetres long. The pale yellow flowers grow from the branches and bear fruits with soft spikes on the skin. The fruits can vary in length from 10-30 centimetres, weigh up to 6.5 kilograms and are full of white pulp with small black seeds.

Parts Used: Leaves; Fruits; Stems; Bark; Seeds

Traditional Uses

Sour sop is used traditionally in Jamaica to treat worms, reduce blood pressure and as a tranquiliser. The leaves, bark and stem of the sour sop tree can be infused or decocted to treat a wide range of health conditions: to calm the nerves, for fevers, coughs and as a general tonic. The bark and leaves are also used in combination with other herbs for conditions such as prostate problems and as key ingredients in some of the popular roots drinks and tonics.

In the Eastern Caribbean the leaves are crushed and inhaled to revive someone from a fainting spell, for dizziness, or to deaden pain. The bark is decocted and taken for dysentery and worms.

Women in labour take a bath in a leaf decoction and drink the tea to help with childbirth, and the tea is also said to increase lactation.

In Central and South America, sour sop has a long history in herbal healing which makes use of almost all parts of the fruit and tree. The fruit is used for worms, to cool fevers, and in cases of diarrhoea. The sour sop leaves, bark and roots are used in some countries in that region to treat a range of health problems, including diabetes, high blood pressure, heart problems, nervous conditions, pain, internal parasites, coughs, flu and difficult childbirth.

Modern Research and Uses

There have been many studies of the active compounds in sour sop, dating back more than 50 years. Most of these studies have focused on a group of compounds called annonaceous acetogenins, which are unique to the annonaceae plant family. These plant chemicals are reported to exhibit significant toxicity to a number of cancer cell lines, and this activity has been reported in both in vitro and in vivo studies. The active plant chemicals in sour sop kill cancer cells without harming healthy ones and have been particularly effective where multi-drug resistant cells have resisted available chemotherapy.

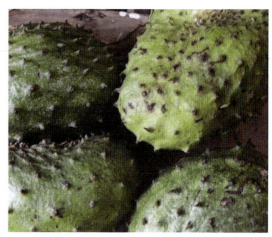

Other studies have confirmed that these active plant chemicals have significant effects on the malaria parasite in animal tests and also demonstrated anti-microbial, antiviral and pesticidal activity. Traditional use of sour sop to treat internal parasites has also been validated by various studies. Research findings have also pointed to the fact that sour sop can lower blood pressure, regulate the nervous system, relieve insomnia and can be helpful in cases of kidney and gall bladder disorders. A recent study of the effects of a water extract of sour sop leaves showed effectiveness in treating jaundice and other liver damage in rats.

Plant Chemicals

Plant chemicals in sour sop include: acetogenins; alkaloids; steroids; flavonoids; terpenoids; saponins; glycosides; phenols; carotenoids; essential oils.

Other Uses

The pulp of the sour sop is used to make a variety of drinks, desserts and confectionery. Milk, sugar or honey, colouring or alcohol can be added to beverages made from sour sop. In many Central and South American and Southeast Asian countries, sour sop is grown on a commercial scale, and the concentrate made from the fruit is exported.

The pounded seeds contain an effective insecticide, particularly against lice and a number of crop pests, including pea aphids. An essential oil made from sour sop leaves has been used successfully against mosquitos and other insects.

Caution!

People taking medication should not use sour sop without the supervision of a health professional. Long-term use can also affect the natural balance of microbes in the gut. Special care must be exercised when using the bark of the sour sop tree due to an alkaloid in the bark extract, which can cause convulsions and other neurological problems if taken in large quantities.

SPANISH NEEDLE – *Bidens pilosa* – Asteracea

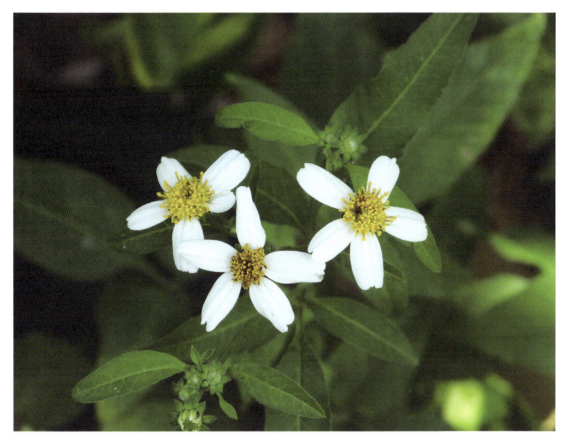

Other Names: Beggar's Tick; Needle Grass; Picao Preto, Z'Herbe Z'Aiguille; Dadayem; Ki Nehe; Acetillo; Blackjack

Brief Description

Spanish needle is a common plant in many tropical and temperate areas growing up to one metre in height. The leaves are about 1-5 centimetres, and the flowers are white with a yellow centre. The brown seeds are like small spikes and fasten to anything that gets near the plant. These spikes are dispersed in the wind or are carried by whatever they attach themselves to, which explains why the plant is so widely distributed.

Parts Used: Leaves; Stems; Flowers; Roots

Traditional Uses

Spanish needle is traditionally used in Jamaica for bowel complaints, cuts, colds, colic and as a de-wormer. The juice is used in the Eastern Caribbean for earaches, inflamed eyes, colds and difficulty in urinating. Spanish needle is used in Cuba for a wide range of illnesses including diabetes, asthma, stomach ulcers, renal infections, menstrual irregularities and as an anti-inflammatory.

In West Africa, spanish needle is used for cuts and wounds as it helps to stop bleeding and promote healing. In different parts of Africa, the juice and tea of the plant is used internally to treat hypertension, malaria, yellow fever, dysentery, diarrhoea, colic and menstrual problems; and externally for rheumatism, skin problems, eye infections and nose bleeds.

Spanish needle is used in South America to combat viruses and bacteria and to inhibit the growth of yeast. It is also reputed to prevent ulcers and lower blood sugar levels. Spanish needle is used in Peru to reduce inflammation and for liver problems. In Brazil, it is used internally for genito-urinary problems, fevers and swellings and as a gargle to treat laryngitis. Spanish needle is applied topically for insect bites, rashes, wounds and fungal infections.

In Polynesia, spanish needle is used to treat urinary tract infections, prostatitis and for liver conditions, such as jaundice and hepatitis. It is regarded as one of the most useful herbs in traditional Chinese medicine for treating a wide variety of health problems including flu, fever, sore throat, acute appendicitis, hepatitis and gastroenteritis, as well as rheumatism, malaria, skin infections, haemorrhoids and insect bites.

Modern Research and Uses

Many traditional uses of spanish needle have been validated by modern research, including its effectiveness as a styptic and for liver problems. Animal and other laboratory tests have also demonstrated that spanish needle has gastro-protective properties and significant antiviral effects, which support its traditional use for colds, flu and respiratory infections. Spanish needle has also been confirmed as having anti-malarial activity in tests on mice and in vitro.

Spanish needle is reported to have anti-microbial and anti-inflammatory properties and in one animal study reduced blood pressure due to its ability to dilate blood vessels. In another study, a chemical cytopiloyne was identified as being key to spanish needle's ability to regulate blood sugar levels. There have also been reports that the plant is effective against the herpes simplex virus, with the hot-water extract proving more potent than other extracts.

A study in China found that a hot-water extract of spanish needle was effective in treating leukaemia, and this anti-leukemic activity has been confirmed by an in vitro study carried out in Japan. A number of other in vitro experiments have reported that plant chemicals in spanish needle have significant anti-tumour and cytotoxic effects on a variety of human cancer cells.

It is clear that spanish needle, which is so widely available, has a lot of potential for a range of health conditions, and there should be further research to ensure that this potential is realised.

Plant Chemicals

Plant chemicals in spanish needle include: phenols; flavonoids; terpenoids; glycosides; steroids; tannins; phenylpropanoids; polyacetylenes; polyynes.

Other Uses

Spanish needle is eaten as a vegetable in some parts of the world, and nutritionists have recommended that the plant should be utilised more due to its high levels of iron, calcium, beta-carotene, zinc and other micro-nutrients. The essential oil from the leaves, flowers and stems of spanish needle has significant therapeutic potential for a range of skin conditions, offering yet more opportunities for economic development.

Spanish needle is commonly used for animal feed.

Caution!

People who are on medication for high blood pressure and diabetes should only use spanish needle internally under the supervision of a health professional to ensure that their blood sugar and blood pressure levels are monitored.

STINKING TOE – *Hymenaea courbaril* – Fabaceae

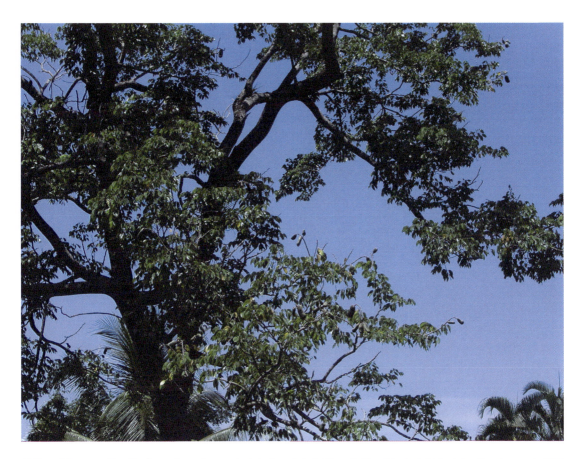

Other Names: South American Locust; Jatoba; Jatai; Copal; Redi Loksi; West Indian Locust; Old Man's Toe; Brazillian Cherry; Rode Locus; Kawanari; Guapinol

Brief Description

The stinking toe tree is native to the forests of South and Central America and the Caribbean. The tree grows up to 40 metres in height and has bright green leaves and white, fragrant flowers that bear an oblong, brown, pod-like fruit with large seeds inside.

Parts Used: Leaves; Fruits; Bark; Resin; Pods

Traditional Uses

Stinking toe is mainly used in Jamaica as a fruit (see below), but in South and Central America and other countries, where the tree grows, it has a long history of medicinal use. The resin which comes from the root of the tree and from the trunk is used to treat upper respiratory tract problems. In Panama, the leaves are used with the bark to treat diabetes, but the bark is the part most widely used. It is used in Suriname to treat urinary tract infections and dysentery. Stinking toe bark extracts either water-based or alcohol-based, are popular in South America as a general tonic for natural energy, to build immunity and to treat a number of health conditions.

Modern Research and Uses

Research on stinking toe began in the 1930s in Brazil, where it was discovered that it was effective in treating a number of disorders and diseases, including dysentery, bronchitis and general fatigue. Most studies on stinking toe have examined the plant chemicals in the bark and resin of the tree, and they have validated many of the traditional uses of the tree parts, in particular its anti-fungal, anti-candida and anti-microbial properties. A study of an extract of the heartwood of the tree showed that it has significant antioxidant activity.

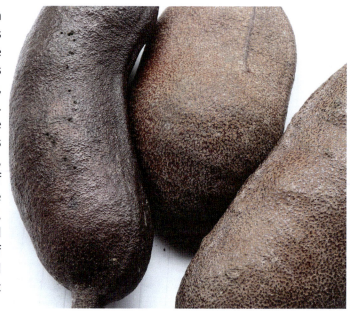

A decoction or tincture of stinking toe bark has been shown in a number of studies to be effective in treating bronchitis, dysentery, diarrhoea, prostatitis, cystitis, urinary tract infections, yeast infections, and fungal infections such as athlete's foot and fungal nail infections. A recent study looking at one of the major constituents of the sap from the stinking toe tree, fisetin, confirmed significant anti-fungal activity as well as cytotoxic effects. This plant chemical, a powerful antioxidant, has now been acknowledged as having benefits in treating prostate cancer, dementia and preventing bone loss.

Plant Chemicals

Plant chemicals in stinking toe include: terpenoids; flavonoids; phenols; steroids; oligosaccharides; tannins.

Other Uses

The stinking toe fruit has a smell that is reflected in its name, but the taste is described as delicious and creamy. The fruit is rich in vitamins B and C and minerals, including calcium, potassium and iron, and can be made into a delicious and nutritious shake with milk or soya. Some people in Jamaica regard stinking toe punch as a powerful drink with medicinal and aphrodisiac properties. In Brazil, the mealy fruit powder is mixed with cassava, maize or flour to make cakes and other baked goods. Stinking toe fruit is high in protein, fibre and micro-nutrients and has potential as a source of nutraceutical products.

The seeds of the fruit can be used to make jewellery, and the pods are used to make craft items. The resin from the root of very old trees is similar to amber and can also be made into jewellery. Lumber from the stinking toe tree has long been prized for its durability and beauty. It is comparable to mahogany and is used for flooring, furniture and construction.

SUSUMBA – *Solanum torvum* – Solanaceae

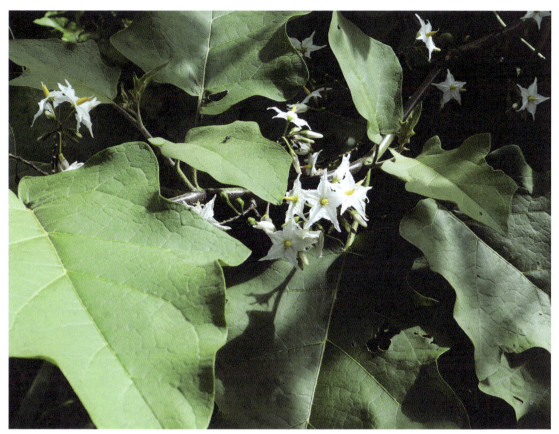

Other Names: Gully Bean; Turkey Berry; Pea Eggplant; Devil's Fig; Melongene Diable; Tandang-aso; Bhurat; Sundakai; Anona Ntroba; Jurubeba; Takakak; Cherry Eggplant

Brief Description

Susumba is native to the Americas but is now found in many tropical regions of the world. It is a spreading shrub which can reach a height of three metres or more. The branches and stems usually have scattered thorns, which are slightly hooked. The leaves, which can range from 10-15 centimetres long and 8-10 centimetres wide, are coarse with small hairs on both sides and mostly seven-lobed, occasionally with smaller thorns. The small white flowers have a yellow centre and bloom in clusters. Fruits are small, round and green, like peas, before turning yellow when ripe.

Parts Used: Fruits; Leaves; Roots

Traditional Uses

Susumba leaf is traditionally used in Jamaica for colds, flu and intestinal parasites, but the fruits are more commonly used as a vegetable (see below). In other countries where susumba grows, the fruits, leaves and roots are used in herbal healing for a wide variety of conditions. In Indian Ayurvedic healing, the roots and fruits are used for urinary retention, kidney stones, stomach disorders and bronchial problems. In some parts of India, susumba is dried, powdered and added to hot water or milk and taken for coughs and colds.

In Ghana, the susumba leaves are used for abdominal pain, and a juice of the uncooked fruits is regarded as beneficial to women after childbirth and to improve their blood. A decoction of the fruits is used there for hypertension and applied topically to treat wounds and various skin infections. A susumba leaf or root poultice is applied to swollen joints in Indonesia and other parts of Asia to reduce swelling and relieve pain. In traditional Chinese medicine, susumba is considered to be effective in blood disorders, swellings and bronchial problems.

Modern Uses and Research

Studies on various parts of the susumba plant have confirmed many of its traditional uses and have discovered a number of new and potentially important ones. One study found that a methanol extract of susumba leaves and fruits had significant anti-microbial effects in both animal and in vitro tests, while another showed that extracts of the dried fruits and the roots are antiviral.

Aqueous extracts of the leaves, on the other hand, had analgesic and anti-inflammatory properties. New compounds discovered in the seeds of the susumba fruits have shown an ability to repair DNA damage and reduce free radicals. At least two studies have suggested that both aqueous and ethanol fruit extracts have anti-hypertensive and blood-thinning properties. One of these studies indicated that this extract exhibited angiotensin-converting enzyme (ACE) inhibiting activity, similar to some anti-hypertensive drugs. Susumba could therefore be very beneficial in a range of cardiac and vascular conditions.

A recent review highlighted the potential benefits of susumba in the treatment of benign prostatic hyperplasia (BPH) which is particularly common in men of African heritage. This is perhaps due to the plant's effects on modulating the immune system as well as its antioxidant and anti-inflammatory properties.

Plant Chemicals

Plant chemicals in susumba include: steroids; phenols; terpenoids; saponins; alkaloids; tannins; flavonoids.

Other Uses

In most places where susumba grows, the fruits are used in a variety of culinary dishes. In India, the fruits are dried, powdered and made into a sauce. Susumba berries are commonly used in Thai green curry and for various other dishes in Southeast Asian recipes. In Jamaica, it is usually cooked with salted codfish and sometimes with ackee. Susumba is rich in micronutrients such as calcium, vitamins B and C, potassium and iron.

The susumba plant is also used as a rootstock for eggplants or aubergines as it is supposed to make them less susceptible to fungal and other diseases.

Caution!

There have been a number of reports of adverse reactions after consuming susumba, but further study needs to be done to establish the underlying causes. It might be advisable to soak the fruits in hot water before cooking. A study carried out in Cuba did not find susumba to be toxic, but another study suggested that there could be differences in the concentration of some of the chemical compounds found in the plant, depending on where it grows.

TRUMPET TREE- *Cecropia peltata* – Cecropiaceae

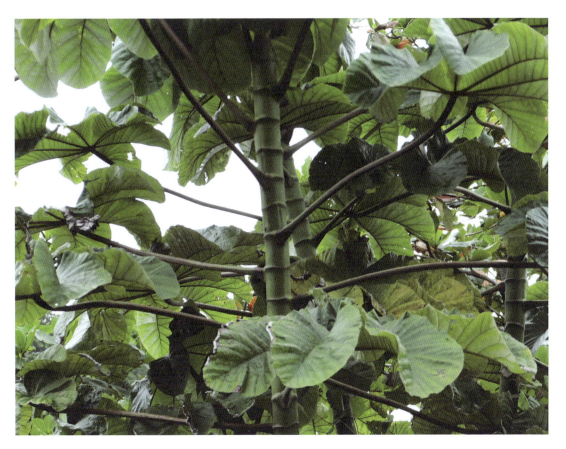

Other Names: Snake Wood Tree; Bois Trompette; Bois Canon; Embauba; Bospapaja; Yagruma; Igarata; Pumpwood

Brief Description

Trumpet tree grows in Central and South America and the Caribbean and can reach up to 20 metres in height. The tree is fast growing, and the trunk is hollow. It has large, lobed leaves which can be up to 30 centimetres in diameter, and bears grey-brown fruits, which are popular with bats.

Parts Used: Leaves; Latex; Bark

Traditional Uses

In Jamaica, trumpet tree is used mainly for colds, sore throat, hoarseness and nerves but is not used as widely today as it once was. In Barbados and Trinidad and Tobago, trumpet leaves are still popular for treating diabetes. There are other uses for the tree parts in Trinidad and Tobago, to treat colds, fever, flu, snake and scorpion bites.

In Cuba and Central America, the latex from the trunk is used to treat warts, corns, calluses, herpes and skin ulcers, and the leaves for asthma. The leaves are also used to treat liver and kidney disorders and to increase menstruation. Trumpet leaves have long been regarded as an effective treatment for diabetes in Mexico and other Central American countries. In South America, as well as using trumpet tree leaves to treat asthma and other upper respiratory tract infections, the leaves are used to treat diabetes, high blood pressure and heart problems. Trumpet tree is also reputed to be effective in treating reproductive problems, menstruation and childbirth.

Modern Research and Uses

Many traditional uses of the trumpet tree have been confirmed by recent clinical research. The ability of trumpet tree to reduce high blood pressure is thought to be the result of ACE-inhibiting activity in some of its plant chemicals. In 2002, a US Patent was taken out on phytochemicals in trumpet tree which are believed to have cardio-tonic and diuretic properties.

Independent research has not yet confirmed the anti-asthmatic activity of trumpet tree leaves. There is, however, evidence to suggest that an alcohol extract of the leaf is active against Staphylococcus aureus. The traditional use of trumpet tree leaves to treat diabetes has been supported by recent experiments in rats. Studies have also confirmed the plant's ability to stem blood flow and its wound-healing properties.

Plant Chemicals

Plant chemicals in trumpet tree include: glycosides; alkaloids; flavonoids; tannins; phenols; steroids; terpenoids.

Other Uses

Trumpet tree is used to make rafts and for boards and palings.

Caution!

People on medication for heart problems, diabetes or blood pressure should not use trumpet tree unless under supervision as the activity of the plants chemicals can increase the activity of the drugs used to treat these conditions. It is not advisable to use trumpet tree in pregnancy!

VERVINE – Stachytarpheta jamaicensis – Verbenaceae

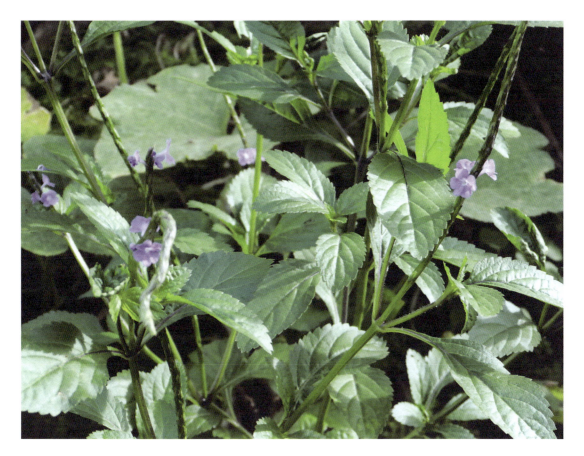

Other Names: Bastard Vervain; Blue Verbena; Rat Tail; Gervao; Rooster Comb; Kandikandilaan; Blue Porterweed; Verveine Queue de Rat; Brazilian Tea

Brief Description

Vervine is native to the tropical Americas, but is now found in Africa, Asia and the Pacific regions. It grows up to one metre high with dark green veined leaves and has bluish, purple flowers, which grow on spikes.

Parts Used: Leaves; Roots; Whole Plant

Traditional Uses

Vervine is used traditionally in Jamaica for nervous disorders, as an eye tonic and to clean wounds. Traditionally, it is combined with sour sop and semi-contract to expel worms and other intestinal parasites. Vervine is also used for a variety of female sexual and reproductive health conditions. In the Eastern Caribbean, vervine is used for colds, fevers, and worms. The leaves are applied to sores and wounds to cleanse and heal.

In Africa, vervine is used to treat menstrual problems and to help contract the uterus after childbirth. It is also believed to be effective for gonorrhoea, eye trouble and heart conditions. Vervine is used in South America for respiratory problems such as asthma, for gastric problems, including ulcers and to treat chronic liver disorders.

In Southeast Asia, they use vervine mainly for a range of gastro-intestinal disorders, including acid reflux, ulcers, intestinal worms and constipation, as well as liver ailments. The plant is also thought to be beneficial for respiratory problems and for skin conditions such as boils, sores and wounds.

Modern Research and Uses

Recent research has confirmed the properties of various plant chemicals in vervine, which validate many of the herb's traditional uses. Vervine has been shown to be effective in treating a variety of gastric disorders including ulcers and diarrhoea. It has anti-inflammatory, antihistamine and pain relieving activity. These effects support traditional use of vervine especially for inflammatory disorders and menstrual problems. Studies have also confirmed the herb's effectiveness in treating respiratory problems such as bronchitis and asthma and as a mild sedative and diuretic.

A recent study in Nigeria demonstrated that water-based extracts from vervine had varying effects on a range of bacteria and microbes. Alcohol-based extracts had activity on fewer organisms, and in another study, the root extract proved to have anti-microbial effects. A study in Spain reported significant antioxidant and immune-stimulating activity in vervine. Research carried out in Jamaica confirmed vervine's effectiveness in treating intestinal parasites.

Documented studies on vervine indicate that this herb has many medicinal properties that could be useful in treating a wide variety of health conditions. Further studies need to be undertaken in order to develop standardised products from this common plant.

Plant Chemicals

Plant chemicals in vervine include: phenols; terpenoids; steroids; saponins; flavonoids; tannins; glycosides; alkaloids; glucosides.

Caution!

A decoction of the roots can induce abortion so should not be used during pregnancy. Care should also be taken if using medication for hypertension and heart problems.

WILD CASSAVA – *Jatropha gossypifolia* – Euphorbiacea

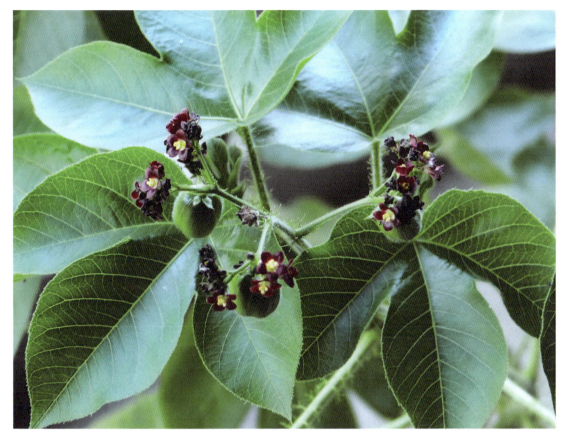

Other Names: Cassava Marble; Bellyache Bush; Wild Physic Nut; Lapalapa; Tuba-tuba; Ratan Jyoti; Pignut; Medicinier Sauvage; Sosori; Frailecillo

Brief Description

Wild cassava is found in many tropical parts of the world, and is related to the physic nut (Jatropha curcas). This shrub grows up to 1.5 metre high, with lobed leaves about ten centimetres long, which often have a purplish tinge. The plant is covered in tiny hairs with deep purple flowers that bear the fruits or 'marbles'.

Parts Used: Leaves; Seeds; Oil; Fruits; Latex

Traditional Uses

In Jamaica and Barbados, wild cassava is traditionally used to treat stomach problems. Wild cassava is reputed to be good for 'stoppage of water' and prostrate health in general. An infusion of the leaves is taken to relieve everything from biliousness and constipation to ulcers. Like physic nut, the fruit can be taken as an emetic or as a purgative depending on the amount ingested. A decoction of wild cassava leaves is used as a blood purifier and as a bath for fevers and skin conditions such as eczema.

Wild cassava leaves can be heated and made into a poultice to relieve painful joints or skin problems such as boils, sores and even leprosy. In Ghana, the leaf juice of the wild cassava is applied to the lining of the mouth and the tongue of children who have oral thrush. It is also used there as an emetic and purgative. In other parts of Africa, the sap or latex of the plant is used to stem blood flow both in cuts and nose bleeds.

Modern Research and Uses

In a study carried out on 30 healthy subjects, the latex of wild cassava was applied to small skin punctures. The bleeding time and the time taken for the blood to clot, with and without the stem latex, were recorded and compared. When the latex was applied, both times were significantly shorter, which supports the traditional use of wild cassava latex as a haemostatic agent. In other studies, a methanol extract of wild cassava leaves was shown to have anti-inflammatory and analgesic activity in experimental animal models. The effects compared well with those of standard non-steroidal anti-inflammatory drugs (NSAIDs) such as diclofenac and indomethacin.

Other studies on animals have reported that wild cassava leaf extracts have significant anti-microbial properties. In a study, rats were given a wild cassava leaf and stem infusion for four weeks; their systolic blood pressure was reduced. Tests carried out on animal tumours and in vitro cancer cells have shown that plant chemicals in wild cassava have potent anti-tumour and cytotoxic activity.

Wild cassava leaf extracts have been reported in two studies in mice as having anti-fertility and abortifacient properties, but more research needs to be done to identify which chemicals are involved in these effects. All these findings suggest that new medicinal products could be derived from the different parts of wild cassava.

Plant Chemicals

Plant chemicals in wild cassava include: alkaloids; tannins; saponins; flavonoids; glycosides; steroids; terpenoids; lignans; coumarins; phenols.

Other Uses

The oil of the wild cassava seeds is still used in some parts of the world for lighting purposes. The need for biofuels worldwide is growing, and as a member of the Jatropha species, commercial production of wild cassava seed oil is set to increase.

In parts of Africa and South America, wild cassava is planted to provide protection from supernatural forces, including bewitchment. It is also believed to protect against snakes and lightning strikes!!

Caution!

There have been some reports of toxicity in wild cassava roots and seeds, although these incidents are rare, it is advisable not to use these parts of the plant internally unless recommended by a health practitioner. Avoid using wild cassava internally if pregnant or trying to become pregnant and if using medication.

WILD COFFEE – *Casearia sylvestris* – Flacourtiaceae

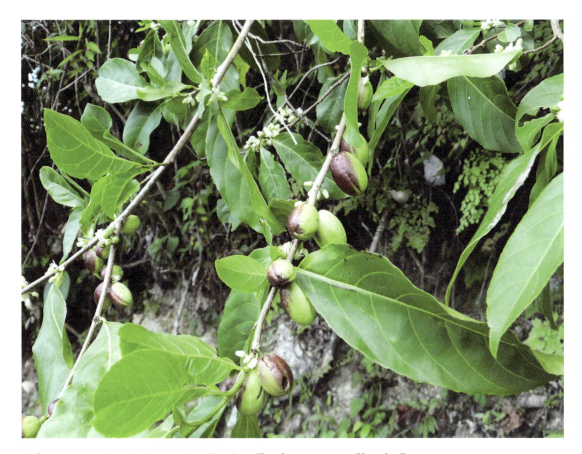

Other Names: Crack Open; Cafeillo; Sarnilla; Guacatonga; Cha-de-Bugre

Brief Description

Wild coffee is native to Central and South America and the Caribbean. It is a small tree, which reaches up to two or three metres, but can be as much as ten metres in height. The leaves are oval, from 5-15 centimetres long, with tiny white, cream or greenish clusters of flowers bearing on a short stalk. The flowers smell like a mixture of honey and urine and bear small fruits, which have three seeds when they 'crack open'.

Parts Used: Leaves; Bark; Roots

Traditional Uses

Wild coffee is not used in Jamaica as a healing agent, but is used in South America, particularly Brazil, Bolivia and Peru, mainly for snake, dog and insect bites. The leaves are used traditionally to treat stomach problems, such as ulcers, diarrhoea, and food poisoning.

Wild coffee is used in parts of South America to purify the blood and for pain relief, and in Bolivia, it is valued for its ability to stop bleeding and reduce infection and inflammation in wounds. Wild coffee is also reputed to be effective in treating a variety of skin problems, including eczema, burns, leprosy and herpes, and is an ingredient in dental mouthwashes.

Modern Research and Uses

In the last 20 years, there have been a number of research projects, which have looked at wild coffee's anti-tumour and anti-cancer properties. Patents were taken out by Japanese researchers on isolated compounds called casearins, to treat various cancers. More recently, previously unknown casearins have been discovered by American researchers, again as anti-cancerous agents.

Most of the research done on wild coffee has been carried out by Brazilians, who have focused mainly on the pain-relieving and anti-ulcer properties of the plant. A very recent study found that wild coffee has significant anti-microbial and anti-fungal activity. Another study demonstrated that extracts of wild coffee leaves have significant anti-inflammatory and antioxidant activity. Wild coffee has also been reported as being effective in lowering lipid levels.

The traditional use of wild coffee for insect and snake bites and as a styptic, has also been borne out by various laboratory tests and animal studies. A recent study concluded that extracts from wild coffee had the best effect against the leishmaniasis protozoa, which cause death and disability in many tropical countries. This underused plant needs further research on its healing properties in order to develop its pharmaceutical potential.

Plant Chemicals

Plant chemicals in wild coffee include: flavonoids; phenols; terpenoids; glycosides; essential oils.

Other Uses

A commercially made perfume in Brazil is based on the essential oil extracted from wild coffee leaves. Wild coffee is also an ingredient in a weight loss product made in Brazil.

Caution!

Due to wild coffee's proven anti-microbial and anti-fungal effects, it would be advisable to ensure that the natural flora in the gut is balanced by eating yoghurt or similar product, if using wild coffee for prolonged periods.

Appendices

How to Use Herbs

Glossary of Medical Terms

Common Health Conditions

Index of Plants – Common Names

Index of Plants – Botanical Names

How to Use Herbs

Many of the books referred to in the **Bibliography** provide more detailed information on the many ways to use herbs. Here, I will give a brief summary of these.

Herbs can be used either fresh or dried, depending on the particular use and herb. It is important that the herb is in good condition, without mould or fungus and free from infestation by insects. Many of the herbs described in this book might be difficult to find fresh in Europe and North America as they are mostly sourced from tropical and sub-tropical regions.

With few exceptions, however, many of the herbs can be obtained over the internet or in health food stores, either in loose form, as tinctures, extracts, tablets/capsules or in creams and other preparations. Whatever the source, it is important to ensure that the source is reputable and as always, when in doubt, ask questions of your suppliers.

Teas (Infusion)

Teas can be made with a single herb or with a combination of herbs. Teas are generally best for those herbs which have active plant chemicals that are water-soluble. Infusions are the best way to prepare delicate parts of plants, such as the leaves and flowers, and for plants which have high levels of essential oils.

To make an infusion, pour boiling water on fresh or dried herbs and leave for 10-15 minutes, strain and drink. The ratio of herb to water varies according to the particular herb and its intended usage, but on average 10-15g (1/2oz) of cut herbs to 500ml (1pt) water. Use less if the herb has been finely cut or powdered. For medicinal use, drink ½-1 cup 2-3 times per day. Infusions can also be used externally for skin problems, minor burns, and sprains (see Compresses below).

Teas (Decoction)

Teas made from roots, bark, berries and twigs are best used as a decoction. The ratio is 20g herb to 500ml (1pt) water. In a decoction, the herb is boiled for 20-30 minutes as the longer time helps to release the active plant chemicals. Some decoctions are boiled for even longer. This is particularly true of tough barks and twigs and ensures that the medicinal content is fully extracted. The dosage can be the same as for infusions; decoctions can also be used externally.

Tinctures

Tinctures are made when the herb is soaked in alcohol or an alcohol/water mix, which can better extract the active plant chemicals from the herb. Tinctures are stronger than infusions and decoctions and can last 1-2 years, depending on the ratio of water to alcohol and proper storage. They are better suited to herbs which have a bitter or unpleasant taste and are also convenient if using while away from home or without access to cooking facilities.

Tinctures can be made with both fresh and dried herbs. For fresh herbs, the ratio is 1 part herb to 2 or 3 parts alcohol, i.e. 300g (12ozs): 1 litre (2pts). When using dried herbs, the ratio is 1 part herb to 4 parts alcohol; 250g (10 ozs): 1 litre alcohol. Some herbalists prefer to use a 1:5 ratio.

The mixture should be stored in a glass jar and left to soak for at least three weeks, shaking the container every couple of days. Strain the mixture, squeezing out as much of the liquid as possible with a muslin cloth or wine press. Store the liquid and use as required. The dosage varies according to the herb and the medicinal need, but is usually about 2-5mls, taken in juice or water, 2-3 times a day.

For people who don't want to consume alcohol or are pregnant, the tincture can be put into a small cup of hot water and left for some minutes for the alcohol to evaporate. Tinctures can also be made using vinegar and glycerine.

Tinctures can also be used externally and can be added to other herbal blends (see below).

Poultices

Poultices are a traditional way of using herbs externally to treat skin problems, sprains and for muscular or nerve pains. The herb can be heated either in hot water or over a low, open flame and applied to the affected area. The herb can be powdered, or mashed up in a mortar and placed between two pieces of cloth and tied onto the body part. This can be left on for up to three hours or as necessary.

Compresses

A herbal mixture made from an infusion, decoction or from a tincture can be used for external problems such as sprains, bruises, inflammations, fevers, or headaches. Compresses are applied by using a cloth soaked in the mixture to the particular part of the body. The mixture can be hot or cold or alternating, depending on the condition.

Glossary of Medical Terms

Abortifacient	- Causes abortions
Adaptogen	- Helps the body adapt to stress and supports normal function
Analgesic	- Reduces pain
Anaesthetic	- Numbs perception of external sensations
Anaphylactic	- Produces extreme allergic reaction
Anthelmintic	- Expels or destroys parasitic worms
Anti-anxiety	- Protects against feelings of intense fear, real or imagined
Antibiotic	- Destroys or inhibits micro-organisms
Anti-candida	- Destroys or inhibits growth of candida yeast infections
Anti-coagulant	- Prevents blood clotting
Antidepressant	- Treats depression
Anti-fungal	- Combats fungal infections
Antihistamine	- Reduces allergic reaction caused by histamine production
Anti-inflammatory	- Reduces inflammation
Anti-malarial	- Destroys organism causing malaria, or used to treat malaria
Anti-microbial	- Destroys or inhibits micro-organisms
Anti-neurasthenic	- Helps to relieve symptoms of neurasthenia, a psychosomatic disorder
Antioxidant	- Prevents oxidation and breakdown of tissues
Anti-periodic	- Prevents regular recurrence of symptoms of a disease
Anti-protozoal	- Destroys protozoal infections
Antiseptic	- Destroys or inhibits infection causing organisms
Anti-spasmodic	- Prevents and relieves muscle spasms
Anti-tetanus	- Destroys bacteria that cause tetanus

Anti-tumorous	- Retards or prevent uncontrolled cell growth
Antitussive	- Soothes and relieves coughing
Anti-ulcerogenic	- Relieves symptoms of gastric and other ulcers
Aphrodisiac	- Excites libido and sexual organs
Astringent	- Tightens mucous membranes and skin, reducing secretions and bleeding
Auto-immune	- Resulting from the immune system attacking the body
Bitter	- Stimulates the appetite
Bronchodilator	- Dilates and relaxes bronchial muscles
Carcinogenic	- Causes cancer
Cardiotonic	- Strengthens the heart and improves heart function
Carminative	- Relieves gas and indigestion
Demulcent	- Soothes and protects body surfaces and mucous
Detoxification	- Removal of toxins and waste from the body
Digestive	- Aids digestion
Diuretic	- Stimulates flow of urine
Edema	- Retention of fluid
Emetic	- Induces vomiting
Emmenagogue	- Causes vomiting
Expectorant	- Helps clear phlegm form the throat and chest
Febrifuge	- Reduces fever
Haemostatic	- Stops or reduces bleeding
Hepatic	- Affects the liver
Hepato-protective	- Protects the liver
Hyperglycaemic	- Raises blood sugar levels
Hypertension	- High blood pressure

Hypoglycaemic   - Lowers blood sugar level

Hypotension   - Low blood pressure

Immune stimulant   - A substance that stimulates the body's immune defences

Immuno-modulator   - A substance capable of modifying or regulating immune functions

Laxative   - Promotes evacuation of the bowels

Narcotic   - Causes drowsiness or stupor and relieve pain

Nervine   - Restores the nerves, relaxes the nervous system

Pectoral   - Relieves disorders of the chest and lungs

Pesticidal   - Destroys insects and other pests

Phytochemical   - A biologically active compound found in plants

Psychotropic   - Affects a person's mental or psychological state

Pulmonary   - Those conditions that affect the lungs

Purgative   - A very strong laxative

Sedative   - Reduces activity and nervous excitement

Stimulant   - Increase activity and nervous excitement

Styptic   - Stops bleeding

Systemic   - Affects the body as a whole

Tonic   - Restores and nourishes the body

Topical   - Applied to any part of the body's surface

Vaso-constrictor   - Contracts and narrows blood vessels

Vaso-dilator   - Relaxes and widens blood vessels

Vermifuge   - Expels intestinal worms

Common Health Conditions

Below is a quick Reference Table about using the herbs included in this book to treat a variety of health conditions. This is not intended to be a substitute for medical treatment or consultation with a health professional and no claims are being made in that regard. In fact the need to seek professional help is stressed throughout the book.

Trained, qualified herbal healers and other health professionals can provide services for people who have any health concerns. For less serious and common ailments, herbs can be useful, if used safely and with the same caution and common sense you would apply to using over the counter drugs.

HEALTH CONDITIONS	HERBS RECOMMENDED
Abscesses / Boils	Leaf of Life, Spanish Needle, Jack'na Bush, Four o' Clock, John Charles, Wild Cassava, Guaco, Dandelion, Oil Nut, Cerassee Four o' Clock, John Charles, Wild Cassava, Guaco, Dandelion, Oil Nut, Cerassee
Anxiety	Passion Fruit, Sour Sop, Christmas Candlestick, Shamy Darling, Guava, Hog Plum
Arthritis/Rheumatoid Arthritis	Leaf of Life, Ramgoat Regular, Guaco, Guinea Hen Weed, Noni, John Charles, Marigoule, Bitter Albut, Pimento, Fatten Barrow, Susumba, Wild Cassava, Christmas Candlestick, Nickel, Oil Nut, Ganja, Pepper Elder
Asthma	Milk Weed, Leaf of Life, Trumpet Tree, Ganja, Vervine
Blood Pressure (Hypertension)	Trumpet Tree, Milk Weed, Bas Cedar, Sour Sop, Carry Mi Seed, Passion Fruit, Moringa, Susumba, Pepper Elder, Hog Plum, Guava, Annatto
Bronchitis	Guaco, Vervine, Guinea Hen Weed, Bas Cedar, Spanish Needle, Stinking Toe, Milk Weed, Trumpet Tree, Leaf of Life
Burns	Annatto, Jack'na Bush, Leaf of Life, Oil Nut, Donkey Peepee, Wild Coffee
Cancer	Sour Sop, Guinea Hen Weed, Wild Coffee, John Charles, Cerassee, Spanish Needle, Pimento, Wild Cassava, Noni, Ganja
Colds	Carry Mi Seed, Bas Cedar, Guinea Hen Weed, John Charles, Guaco, Spanish Needle, Passion Fruit, Leaf of Life, Christmas Candlestick, Fatten Barrow, Sage, Moringa, Noni, Stinking Toe
Convulsions (Fits)	Fatten Barrow, Sour Sop, Donkey Peepee, Hog Plum, Christmas Candlestick, Passion Fruit, Ganja, Shamy Darling
Cuts/Wounds	Spanish Needle, Jack'na Bush, Sage, Wild Cassava, Bas Cedar, Marigoule, Wild Coffee, Hog Plum, Trumpet Tree, Guava, Donkey Peepee, Christmas Candlestick, Vervine

Cystitis	Stinking Toe, Annatto, Guinea Hen Weed, Carry Mi Seed, Spanish Needle
Dermatitis/Eczema	John Charles, Moringa, Sage, Guaco, Dandelion, Cerassee, Spanish Needle, Four o' Clock, Fatten Barrow, Wild Coffee, Wild Cassava, King of the Forest, Oil Nut
Detoxification	Bitter Albut, Dandelion, Moringa, Carry Mi Seed, King of the Forest, Cerassee, Vervine, John Charles, Spanish Needle
Diabetes	Queen's Flower, Marigoule, Spanish Needle, Nickel, Cerassee, Trumpet Tree, Bitter Albut, Christmas Candlestick, Annatto, King of the Forest, Ramgoat Regular
Diarrhoea	Guava, Stinking Toe, Fatten Barrow, Hog Plum, Christmas Candlestick, Cerassee, Bitter Albut, Sage, John Charles, Sour Sop, Bas Cedar, Spanish Needle
Digestive Disorders	Wild Cassava, Pimento, Ramgoat Regular, Guaco Cerassee, Donkey Peepee, Vervine, Wild Coffee, Pepper Elder, Annatto, Ganja
Fever	Carry Mi Seed, Nickel, Bitter Albut, Leaf of Life, Marigoule, Spanish Needle, Sage, Annatto, Donkey Peepee
Flu	Guinea Hen Weed, John Charles, Carry Mi Seed, Spanish Needle, Noni, Moringa, Leaf of Life, Four o' Clock, John Charles, Wild Cassava, Guaco, Dandelion, Oil Nut, Cerassee
Fungal Infections	Stinking Toe, King of the Forest, Dandelion, John Charles, Guaco, Oil Nut
Haemorrhoids	Jack'na Bush, Cerassee, Shamy Darling, Spanish Needle, Wild Cassava, Trumpet Tree
Immune Function	Noni, Dandelion, Leaf of Life, Vervine, Susumba Cerassee, Nickel, Guinea Hen Weed
Kidney Problems	Carry Mi Seed, Dandelion, Donkey Peepee, Sour Sop, Passion Fruit, Pepper Elder
Laxative/Purgative	King of the Forest, Oil Nut, Moringa, Wild Cassava, Queen's Flower,
Liver Disorders	Carry Mi Seed, Spanish Needle, Dandelion, Annatto, Christmas Candlestick
Malaria	Sage, Hog Plum, Bitter Albut, Carry Mi Seed, Nickel, Dandelion, Spanish Needle
Menstrual Disorders	Hog Plum, Vervine, Marigoule, Passion Fruit, Shamy Darling, Pimento, Ganja, Christmas Candlestick, Guava,
Nausea/Vomiting	Pepper Elder, Ganja, Sage
Neurological Disorders	Christmas Candlestick, Hog Plum, Shamy Darling, Passion Fruit, Fatten Barrow, Sour Sop, Ganja, Vervine, Guava
Pain Relief	Carry Mi Seed, Wild Cassava, Ganja, Guaco, Guinea Hen Weed, Passion Fruit, Pimento, Leaf of Life, Guava, Noni, Bitter Albut, Wild Coffee, Marigoule, Fatten Barrow

Prostate Problems	Guinea Hen Weed, Carry Mi Seed, Spanish Needle, Stinking Toe, Susumba, Pimento, Annatto
Ringworm	King of the Forest, Stinking Toe, Cerassee, Dandelion, John Charles, Bitter Albut
Sexually Transmitted Infections	Carry Mi Seed, Hog Plum, Spanish Needle, King of the Forest, Bas Cedar, Marigoule
Skin Problems	King of the Forest, Cerassee, John Charles, Guaco, Jack'na Bush, Guinea Hen Weed, Four o' Clock, Moringa, Spanish Needle, Fatten Barrow, Dandelion, Donkey Peepee, Wild Coffee, Sage, Hog Plum, Bitter Albut
Stings/Bites	Leaf of Life, Guaco, King of the Forest, Wild Coffee, Spanish Needle, Vervine, Four o' Clock
Styptic (stops bleeding)	Spanish Needle, Jack'na Bush, Wild Cassava, Wild Coffee,
Toothache/Gum Problems	Sage, Guava, Pimento, Wild Coffee
Ulcers (gastric)	Ramgoat Regular, Wild Coffee, Annatto, Moringa, Vervine, Spanish Needle, Sage, John Charles
Ulcers (sores)	Jack'na Bush, Bitter Albut, Sage, Guava, Hog Plum, John Charles, Trumpet Tree, Bas Cedar, Susumba, Vervine, Fatten Barrow, Donkey Peepee
Urinary Tract Disorders	Carry Mi Seed, Guinea Hen Weed, Stinking Toe, Spanish Needle, Annatto, Moringa
Uterine Bleeding/Fibroids	Shamy Darling, Hog Plum, Bitter Albut, Wild Coffee, Bas Cedar, Marigoule
Worms/Intestinal Parasites	Sour Sop, Vervine, Hog Plum, Four o' Clock, Bitter Albut

Index of Plants – Common Names

Index of Plants – Botanical Names

References

Research Studies

Morrison, E. (1994). Local Remedies -Yeh or Nay. West Indian Med J, 43 (Suppl2), pp. 999-103

Mitchell, S and Ahmad, M. (2006). A Review of Medicinal Plant Research at the University of the West Indies, Jamaica 1948-2001. WI Med J, 55(4), pp. 243-269

Huaman, O et al. (2009). Antiulcer effect of lyophilized hydroalcoholic extract of Bixa orellana (annatto) leaves in rats. Annals of the Faculty of Medicine, vol 70 (2), pp. 97-102

Russell, KR et al. (2005). The effect of annatto on insulin binding properties in the dog. Phytother Res. May 19(5), pp. 433-6

Yong, Y et al. (2013). Chemical constituents and antihistamine activity of Bixa Orellana leaf extract. BMC Complementary and Alternative Medicine. 13:32. doi:10.1186/1472-6882-13-32

Fleischer, TC et al. (2003). Antimicrobial activity of the leaves and seeds from Bixa Orellana. Fitoterapia. 74, pp.136-138

Pierpaoli, E et al. (2013). Effect of annatto- tocotrienols supplementation in the development of mammary tumors in HER-2/neu transgenic mice. Carcinogenesis. doi:10.1093/carcin/bgt 064

Sasikumar, J et al. (2012). Studies on in vitro free radical scavenging activity of Bixa Orellana L. bark extract. Int J Pharm Pharm Sci. vol 4 (2), pp. 719-726

Frega, N et al. (1998). Identification and estimation of tocotrienols in the annatto lipid fraction by gas chromatography mass spectrometry. JAOCS. vol.75 (12), pp 1723-1726

Rojas, J et al. (2006). Screening for Anti-microbial Activity of Ten Medicinal Plants Used in Colombian Folkloric Medicine: A Possible Alternative Treatment of Non-nosomical Infections. BMC Complementary & Alternative Medicine. 6:2, doi: 10.1186/1472-6882-6-2

De Araújo Vilar, D et al. (2014). Traditional Uses, Chemical Constituents, and Biological Activities of Bixa orellana L.: A Review. The Scientific World Journal. http://dx.doi.org/10.1155/2014/857292

Berenguer, B et al. (2007). The Aerial Parts of Guazuma Ulmifolia Lam. Protects against NSAID Induced Lesions. Journal of Ethnopharmacology. Nov, vol. 114:2, pp. 153-60

Magos GA et al. (2008). Hypotensive and vasorelaxant effects of the procyanidin fraction from Guazuma ulmifolia bark in mormotensive and hypertensive rats. J Ethnopharmacol. April 17; 117(1), pp.58-68

Alonso-Castro, A and Salazar-Olivio, L. (2008). The anti-diabetic properties of Guazuma ulmifolia are mediated by the stimulation of glucose uptake in normal and diabetic adipocytes without inducing adipogenesis. J Ethnopharmacol. July 23, 118 (2), pp. 252-6

Gracioso, J et al. (1998). Antinociceptive effect in mice of a hydroalcoholic extract of Neurolaena lobata (L) R.BR and its organic fractions. J Pharm. Pharmacol. Dec, 50(12), pp.1425-9

Garcia-Gonzalez, M et al. (2007). Anti-pyretic effect of the aqueous extract obtained from leaves of Neurolaena lobata (Asteracea) on a pyretic model induced by Brewer's Yeast. www.revistamedica.ucr.ac vol.1 no.1 (3)

Berger, I et al. (2001). Antiprotozoal activity of Neurolaena lobata. Phytother. Res. June;15 (4), pp. 327-30

Lajter,I et al. (2014). Sesquiterpenes from Neurolaeana lobata and Their Anti-proliferative and Anti-inflammatory Activities. Journal of Natural Products, 77 (3), pp. 576-582

Unger, C et al. (2013). The dichloromethane extract of the ethnomedcial plant Neurolaena lobata inhibits NPM/ALK expression which is causal for anaplastic large cell lymphomagenesis. Intl Journal Oncology. vol. 42 (1), pp. 338-348

Asprey, G and Thornton, P (1953-1955). Medicinal Plants of Jamaica Parts 1-4. West Indian Journal of Medicine. vol. 2-4

Chandra, R. (2000). Lipid Lowering Activity of Phyllanthus niruri. Journal of Medicinal & Aromatic Plant Sciences. 22(1), pp. 29-30

Naik, A and Juvekar R. (2003). Effects of alkaloidal extract of Phyllanthus Niruri on HIV replication. Indian J Med Sci. 57, pp. 387-93

Rashmi, M (2011). Antimicrobial effect of Phyllanthus niruri on Human Pathogenic Microorganisms. www.ijddhrjournal.com October – December; 1(4), pp. 234-238

Ekwenye, U and Njoku, N. (2006). Antibacterial effect of Phyllanthus niruri (chanca piedra) on Three Enteropathogens in Man. Intl.J.Mol.Med.Adv.Sci. 2(2), pp. 184-189

Boim, M et al. (2010). Phyllanthus niruri as a promising alternative treatment for nephrolithiasis. Intl.Braz.J. Urol. Nov-Dec, vol 36(6), pp. 657-664

Samali, A et al. (2012). Evaluation of chemical constituents of Phyllanthus niruri. Afr.J.Pharm. Pharmacol. January, vol.6 (3), pp.125-128

Nerurkar, P et al. (2010). Bitter melon (Momordica charantia) inhibits primary human adipocyte differentiation by modulating adipogenic genes. BMC Complementary and Alternative Medicine. 10:34

Ray, R et al. (2010). Bitter melon (Momordica charantia) extract inhibits breast cancer cell proliferation by modulating cell cycle regulatory genes and promotes apoptosis. Cancer Res. March 1, 70(5), pp.1925-31

Paul, A and Raychaudhuri, S. (2010).Medicinal Uses and Molecular Identification of two Momordica charantia varieties – A Review. eJBio vol.6(2), pp. 43-51

Imran, S et al. (2012). Phytochemical Analysis of Leonotis nepetifolia (L) R.BR. A wild medicinal plant of Lamiaceae. Bioscience Discovery. June 3(2), pp.197-199

Pushpan, R et al. (2012). Ethno-medicinal claims of Leonotis nepetifolia (L) R.BR: A Review. IJRAP. Nov-Dec, 3(6), pp. 783-785

Sobolewska, D et al. (2012). Preliminary Phytochemical and Biological Screening of Methanolic and Acetone Extracts from Leonotis nepetifolia (L) R. BR J Medicinal Plants Research. August, vol.6 (30), pp.4582-85

Oliveira, D et al. (2015). Antibacterial mode of action of the hydroethanolic extract of Leonotis nepetifolia (L) R.Br involves bacterial membrane perturbations. J Ethnopharmacol. Aug, 172, pp.356-363. doi:10.1016/j.jep.2015.06.027

Vasuki, K et al. (2015). Pharmacological properties of Leonotis nepetifolia (L) R.Br – A Short Review. AYUSHDHARA. 2(3), pp.162-166

Yadav, J et al. (2010). Cassia occidentalis: a review of its ethnobotany, phytochemical and pharmacological profile. Fitoterapia . June, 81(4), pp. 223-230

Bhagat, M and Saxena, A. (2010). Evaluation of Cassia occidentalis for in vitro cytoxicity against human cancer cell lines and anti-bacterial activity. Indian J. Pharmacol. August, 42(4), pp. 234-237

Sini, K et al. (2011). Analgesic and anti-pyretic activity of Cassia occidentalis Linn. Annals of Biological Researc. 2(1), pp. 195-200

Onakpa, M and Ajagbonna, O. (2012). Anti-diabetic potentials of Cassia occidenatlis leaf extract on alloxan-induced diabetic albino mice. Int J Pharm Tech Research. vol4 (4), pp. 1766-1769

Amusan, O et al. (1996). Antimalarial active principles of Spathodea campanulata. http://opendocs.ids.ac.uk/opendocs/handle/123456789/11445

Akharaiyi, F et al. (2012). Antibacterial, Phytochemical and Antioxidant Activities of the Leaf Extracts of Gliricidia sepium and Spathodea campanulata. World Applied Sciences Journal. 16(4), pp.523-530

Kowti, R et al. (2010). Antimicrobial activity of ethanol extract of leaf and flower of Spathodea camapanulata P. Beauv. RJPBCS. July-Sept, vol 1(3), pp. 691-698

Heim,S et al. (2012). Antioxidant Activity of Spathodea campanulata (Bignoneaceae) Extracts. Rev Bras Pl Med Botucatu. vol 14(2, pp. 387-392

Ilodigwe, E and Akah, P. (2009). Spathodea camapanulata: An Experimental Evaluation of the Analgesic and Anti-inflammatory Properties of a Traditional Remedy. Asian J Med Sci. September, 1(2), pp. 35-38

Amoateng, P et al. (2012). Anti-convulsant and related neuropharmacological effects of the whole plant extract of Synedrella nodiflora (L) Gaertn. (Asteraceae). Journal of BioAllied Sciences. vol 4(20), pp. 140-148

Bhogaonkar, PY et al. (2011). Pharmacognostic Studies and Antimicrobial Activity of Synedrella nodiflora (L.) Gaertn. BioScience Discovery. July (2) 3, pp. 317-321

Ghosh, R et al. (2013). Pharmacognostic, Phytochemical and Biological Studies of Synedrella nodiflora – A Review. IRJIPS. September vol 1(3), pp. 1-4

Devi, SL et al. (2011). Pharmacognostical and Phytochemical Studies of Mirabilis jalapa Linn. South Asian J of Bio Sciences. September 1(1), pp. 1-6

Oladunmoye, M. (2012). Antioxidant, Free Radical Scavenging Capacity and Antimicrobial Activities of Mirabilis jalapa. J Medicinal Plant Research. April, 6(15), pp. 2909-13

Shaik, S et al. (2012). Phytochemical and Pharmacological Studies of Mirabilis jalapa Linn. Int J Pharmacy & Technology. July; 4 (2), pp. 2075-2084

Zachariah, S et al. (2011). In vitro Antioxidant Potential of Methanolic Extracts of Mirabilis jalapa Linn. Free Radicals and Antioxidants. vol1(4), pp. 82-86

Zachariah, S et al. (2012). In vitro Anthelmintic Activity of Aerial Parts of Mirabilis jalapa Linn. Intl Pharm Sci Rev & Res. Feb, vol 12(1), pp. 107-110

Akanji, O et al. (2016). The antimalarial effect of Momordica charantia L. and Mirabilis jalapa leaf extracts using animal model. JMPR. vol10(24), pp. 344-350. doi: 10.5897/JMPR2016.6046

Leung, L. (2011). Cannabis sativa and its derivatives: Review of medical use. J.Am Board Fam Med. 24, pp. 452-462

Mascolo, N. (2000). Medical Uses and Toxological Profile of Cannabis. Pharmacy and Pharmacological Communications. June, vol.6 (6), pp. 231-234

Fernandez-Ruiz, J et al. (2013). Cannabidiol for neurodegenerative disorders: important new clinical applications for this phytocannabinoid? Br J Clin Pharmacol. Feb, 75(2), pp. 323-333

Christelle, M et al. (2016). Cannabis sativa: The Plant of the Thousand and One Molecules. Front Plant Sci. 7:19. doi: 10.3389/fpls.2016.00019

Lentz, D et al. (1998). Antimicrobial properties of Honduran medicinal plants. Journal of Ethnopharmacology. vol.63 (3) Dec, pp. 253-263

Perez-Amador, M et al. (2010). Phytochemical and Pharmacological Studies on Mikania micrantha HBK (Asteraceae). FYTON. 79, pp. 77-80

Li, Y et al. (2013). Antimicrobial constituents of the leaves of Mikania micrantha H.B.K. PLoS One. Oct 2.doi: 10.1371/journal.pone.0076725

Guttierez, R et al. (2008). Guajava: A review of its traditional uses, phytochemistry and pharmacology. Journal of Ethnopharmacology. April 17, 117(1), pp. 1-27

Ojewole, J. (2005). Hypoglycemic and hypotensive effects of Psydium guajava Linn. (Myrtaceae) leaf aqueous extract. Methods Find Exp Clin Pharmacol. Dec, 27 (10), pp.689-95

Ojewole, J. (2006). Antiinflammatory and analgesic effects of Psidium guajava Linn.(Myrtaceae) leaf aqueous extract in rats and mice. Methods Find Exp Clin Pharmacol. Sept, 287(7), pp. 441-6

Metwally, A et al. (2010). Phytochemical investigations and antimicrobial activity of Psydium guajava L. leaves. Phramacogn Mag. July-Sept, 6(23), pp. 212-218

Barbalho, S et al. (2012). Psidium guajava (Guava): A plant of multipurpose medicinal applications. Med Aromat Plants. 1:4, http://dx.doi.org/10.4172/2167-0412.1000104

Uruena, C et al. (2008). Petiveria alliacea extracts uses multiple mechanisms to inhibit growth of human and mouse tumoral cells. BMC Complementary and Alternative Medicine. 8:60, doi:10.1186/1472-6882-8-60

Kim, S et al. (2006). Antibacterial and antifungal activity of sulphur-containing compounds from Petiveria alliacea L. Journal of Ethnopharmacology. 104, pp. 188-192

Williams, L et al. (2007). A critical review of the therapeutic potential of dibenzyl trisulphide, isolated from Petiveria alliacea L (guinea hen weed, anamu). West Indian Med Journal. Jan, 56 (1), pp. 17-21

Lopes-Martins, R et al. (2002). The anti-inflammatory and analgesic effects of a crude extract of Petiveria alliacea L.(Phytolaccaceae). Phytomedicine. vol 9(3), pp.245-248

Vincenti Perez, A. (2015). Benzyl Trisulphide extract from Petiveria alliacea to suppress SLE manifestations – RISE Program www.slideshare.net/andreacarolinavincenti/benzyl-trisulphide-extract-from-petiveria-a...

Abo, K et al. (1999). Antimicrobial potential of Spondias Mombin, Croton Zambesicus and Zygotritonia Crocea. Phytother Res. Sep,13(6), pp. 494-497

Adediwur, F and Abo, K. (2009). Anti-diabetic Activity of Spondias Mombin Extract in NIDDM Rats. Pharmaceutical Biology. vol.47 (3, pp. 215-218

Ayoka, A et al. (2006). Sedative, Anti-epileptic and Anti-psychotic effects of Spondias Mombin in mice and rats. J.Ethnopharmacol. Jan 1, 103(2), pp. 166-175

Ayoka, A et al. (2008). Medicinal and Economic Value of Spondias mombin. Af J Biomed Res. vol.11, pp.129-136

Idu, M et al. (2002). Studies on the nutritional value and anti-tumour property of the bark of Spondias Mombin. Jnl Med & Biomed Res. 1(2), pp. 46-60

Olugbuyiro, J et al. (2009). AntiMtb activity of triterpenoid-rich fractions from Spondias mombin L. African J Biotech. vol 8 (9), pp. 1807-1809

Akinmoladun, A et al. (2010). Ramipril-like activity of Spondias mombin Linn. against no-flow ischaemia and isoproterenol-induced cardiotoxicity in rat heart. Cardiovascular Toxicology. Dec, 4, pp. 295-305

Amatya, S and Tuladhar, S. (2005). Eupatoric Acid : A novel triterpene from Eupatorium Odoratum. Z.Naturforsch. 60b, pp. 1006-1011

Amatya, S and Tuladhar, S. (2011). In vitro antioxidant activity of extracts from Eupatorium odoratum L. Research Journal of Medicinal Plant. 5 (1), pp. 79-84

Phan, T et al. (1996). An aqueous extract of the leaves of Eupatorium Odoratum (Eupolin) inhibits hydrated collagen lattice contraction by normal human dermal fibroblast. J Altern Complement Med. Fall, 2 (3), pp. 335-343

Wongkrajang, M et al. (1990). Eupatorium Odoratum: An enhancer of hemostasis. Mahidol Jrnl of Pharmaceutical Sciences. Jan-Jun, 17(1), pp. 9-13

Anyasor, G et al. (2011). Phytochemical constituent, proximate analysis, antioxidant, antibacterial and wound-healing properties of leaf extracts of Chromolaena odorata. Annals of Biological Research. 2(2), pp. 441-451

Nwinuka, N et al. (2009). Nutritional and potential medical value of Chromolaena odorata leaves. Int J Trop Ag FS. http://dx.doi.org/10.4314/ijotafs.v3i2.50044

Picking, D et al. (2013). Hyptis verticillata Jacq.: A review of its traditional uses, phytochemistry,, pharmacology and toxicology. Journal of Ethnopharmacology. vol 147(1), pp. 16-41

White, Y et al. (2012). Novel cytotoxic isolated from Jamaican Hyptis verticillata Jacq. Induces apoptosis and overcomes multi-drug resistance. Anticancer Res. Dec, 31(12), pp. 4251-7

Hamada, T et al. (2012). The bioassay-guided isolation of growth inhibitors of Adult T-cell leukemia (ATL); from the Jamaican plant Hyptis verticillata and NMR characterization of hyptoside. Molecules. 17(8), pp. 931-938

Thamlikitkul, V et al. (1990). Randomized controlled trial of Cassia alata for constipation. J Med Assoc Thailand. Apr; 73(4), pp. 217-222

Moriyama, H et al. (2003). Anti-inflammatory activity of heat-treated Cassia alata leaf extract and its flavonoid glycoside. Yakugaku Zasshi. 123(7), pp. 607-611

Moriyama, H et al. (2003). Adenine, an inhibitor of platelet aggregation, from leaves of Cassia alata. Biol Pharm Bull. Sep, 26 (9), pp. 1361-4

Somchit, M and Reezal, I. (2003). In vitro anti-microbial activity of ethanol and water extracts of Cassia alata. J Ethnopharmacology. vol 84(1), pp. 1-4

Idu, M et al. (2006). Preliminary investigation in the phytochemistry and antimicrobial activity of Senna alata leaves. J Applied Sciences. 6 (11), pp. 2481-2485

Sule, WF et al. (2011). Phytochemical properties and in vitro antifungal activity of Senna alata Linn. Crude stem bark extract. J Med Plant Res. vol 5 (2), pp. 176-183

Kamboj, A and Saluja, A.(2009). Bryophyllum pinnatum (Lam) Kurz: Phytochemical and pharmacological profile: A review. Phcog Rev. 3, pp. 364-74

Akinpelu, D. (2000). Antimicrobial activity of Bryophyllum pinnata leaves. Fitoterapia. vol 71 (2), pp. 193-4

Ojewole, J. (2005). Antinociceptive, anti-inflammatory and anti-diabetic effects of Bryophyllum pinnatum (Crassulaceae) leaf aqueous extract. Journal of Ethnopharmacology. May, 99 (1), pp. 9-13

Pattewar, S. (2012). Kalanchoe pinnata: Phytochemical and pharmacological profile. IJPSR. vol 3 (4), pp. 993-1000

Mahata, S et al. (2012). Anticancer property of Bryophyllum pinnata (Lam.) Oken. leaf on human cervical cancer cells. BMC Complementary and Alternative Medicine. 12:15. doi: 10.1186/1472-6882-12-15

Balekar, N et al. (2014). Weledia trilobata L: A Phytochemical and Pharmacological Review. Chiang Mai J Sci. 41(3), pp. 590-605

Kade, I et al. (2010). Aqueous extracts of Sphagneticola trilobata attenuates streptozocin-induced hyperglycaemia in rat models by modulating oxidative stress parameters. Biology and Medicine. 2 (3), pp. 1-13

Toppo, K et al. (2013). Antimicrobial Activity of Sphagneticola trilobata (l) Pruski, Against Some Human Pathogenic Bacteria and Fungi. The Bioscan. 8(2), pp. 695-700

Williams, L et al. (1997). Angiotensin Converting Enzyme inhibiting and anti-dipsogenic activities of Euphorbia hirta extracts. Phytother Res. 11, pp. 401-2

Johnson, P et al. (1999). Euphorbia hirta leaf extracts increase urine output and electrolytes in rats. J Ethnopharmacol. April, 65 (1), pp. 63-69

Patel, S et al. (2009). Review of Phytochemistry and Pharmacological aspects of Euphorbia hirta Linn. JPRHC. vol 1(1), pp. 113-133

Kumar, S et al. (2010). Euphorbia hirta: Its chemistry, traditional and medicinal uses and pharmacological activities. Phcog Rev. 4, pp. 58-61

Fahey, J. (2005). Moringa oleifera: A review of the medical evidence for its nutritional, therapeutic and prophylactic properties. Part 1. Trees for Life Journal 1:5 www.tfljournal.org/article.php/20051201124931586

Atawodi, S et al. (2010). Evaluation of the polyphenol content and antioxidant properties of methanol extracts of the leaves, skin and root bark of Moringa oleifera Lam. J. Med Food. June, 13 (3), pp. 710-16 http://www.mskcc.org/cancer-care/herb/moringa-oleifera#field-herb-research-evidence

Anwar, F et al. (2007). Moringa oleifera: a food plant with multiple medicinal uses. Phytother Res. Ja, 21 (1), pp. 17-25

Ndiaye, M et al. (2002). Contribution to the study of the anti-inflammatory activity of Moringa oleifera (Moringaceae). 47 (2), pp. 201-2

Omotesho K et al. (2013). The potential of moringa tree for poverty alleviation and rural development: Review of evidences on usage and efficacy. International Journal of Development and Sustainability. vol 2 (2), pp. 799-813

Orwa C et al (2009). Agroforestree Database:a tree reference and selection guide version 4.0. http://www.worldagroforestry.org/sites/treedbs/treedatabases.asp

Archana, P et al. (2005). Antipyretic and analgesic activities of Caesalpinia bonducella seed kernel extract. Phytotherapy Res. August, 19 (5), pp. 376-381

Chakrabarti, S et al. (2005). Antidiabetic activity of Caesalpinia bonducella F. in chronic type 2 diabetic model in Long-Evans rats and evaluation of insulin secretagogue property of its fractions on isolated islets. J Ethnopharm. Feb, vol 97(1), pp. 117-122

Gupta, M et al. (2004). Antitumour activity and anti-oxidant status of Caesalpinia bonducella against Ehrlich ascites carcinoma in Swiss albino rats. J Pharmacol Sci. Feb, 94(2), pp. 177-81

Innocent, E et al. (2009). Screening of Traditionally Used Plants for in vivo Antimalarial Activity in Mice. Afr J Trad Complement Altern Med. 6(2), pp.163-167

Shukla, S et al. (2010). In vivo immunomodulatory activities of the aqueous extract of bonduc nut Caesalpinia bonducella seeds. Pharmaceutical Biology. vol 48 (2), pp. 227-230

Singh, V and Raghav, P. (2012). Review on pharmacological properties of Caesalpinia bonduc. L. Int J Med Arom Plants. Sept, vol 2 (3), pp. 524-530

Wang, M and Su, C. (2001). Cancer preventive effect of Morinda citrifolia (Noni). Ann NY Acad Sci. Dec, 952, pp. 161-8

Wang, M et al.. (2002) Morinda citrifolia(Noni): A literature review and recent advances in Noni research. Acta Pharmacol Sin. Dec, 23(12), pp.1127-1141

Brown, A. (2012). Anticancer activity of Morinda citrifolia (Noni) fruit: A review. Phytother Res. Oct, 26 (10), pp. 427-40

Rasal, V et al. (2008). Wound-healing and antioxidant activities of Morinda citrifolia leaf extract in rats. IJPT. 7, pp. 49-52

Singh, D. (2012). Morinda citrifolia L (Noni): A review of the scientific validation for its nutritional and therapeutic properties. 3 (6), pp. 77-91

Nayak, B et al (2011). Hypoglycemic and hepaprotective activity of fermented fruit juice of Morinda citrifolia (Noni) in diabetic rats. Evidence-Based Complementary and Alternative Medicine. Sept, 5 pages. http://dx.doi.org/10.1155/2011/875293

Jena, J and Gupta, A. (2012). Ricinus communis Linn.: A phyto-pharmacologic review. Int J Pharm Pharm Sci. vol 4 (14), pp. 25-29

Naz, R and Bano, A. (2012). Antimicrobial potential of Ricinus communis leaf extracts in different solvents against pathogenic bacterial and fungal strains. Asian Pac J Trop Biomed. 2(12), pp. 944-47

Rana, M et al. (2012). Ricinus communis L – A Review". Int J Pharm Tech Res. 4 (4), pp. 1706-11 www.hort.purdue.edu/newcrop/duke/ricinus communis

Bhakta, S and Das, S. (2015). In praise of the medicinal plant Ricinus communis L: A Review. Global J Res Med Plants & Indigen Med. vol 4(5), pp. 95-105

Barbosa, P et al. (2008). The aqueous extracts of Passiflora alata and Passiflora edulis reduce anxiety-related behaviour without affecting memory process in rats. J Med Food. June, 11(2), pp. 282-8

Sunitha, M and Devaki, K. (2009). Antioxidant activity of Passiflora edulis Sims leaves. Indian J Pharm Sci. May-Jun, 71(3), pp. 310-311

Barbalho, S et al. (2012). Yellow passion fruit rind (Passiflora edulis): An industrial waste or an adjuvant in the maintenance of glycemia and prevention of dyslipidemia? www.hoajonline.com/jdrcm/2050-0866/1/5

Ichimura, T et al. (2006). Anti-hypertensive effect of an extract of Passiflora edulis rind in spontaneously hypertensive rats". Biosci Biotechnol Biochem. March, 70 (3), pp. 718-721

Restrepo, R et al. (2013). Angiotensin Converting Enzyme inhibitory activity of Passiflora edulis f. flavicarpa and Petroselinum crispum (Mill) Fuss. Brit Journal of Pharmaceutical Res. 3 (4), pp. 776-785

Simeone, M et al.(2011). Chemical composition of essential oils from ripe and unripe fruits of Piper amalago L. var.medium (Jacq) Yunck and Piper hispidium sw. Journal of Essential Oil Research vol.23 (5), pp. 54-58

Jacobs, H et al. (1999). Amides of Piper amalago var nigrinodum. Journal of Indian Chemical Society. vol 76, pp. 713-17

Carrara, V et al. (2010). Chemical composition and anti-fungal activity of the essential oil from Piper amalago. Lat Am J Pharm. 29 (8), pp.1459-62

Da Silva Mota, J et al. (2013). Identification of the Volatile Compounds of Leaf, Flower, Root and Stem Oils of Piper amalago (Piperaceae). J Essentl Oil bearing Plants. 16(1), pp. 11-16

Noveas, A et al. (2014). Diuretic and antilithiasic activities of ethanolic extract from Piper amalago (Piperaceae). Phytomedicine. Mar 15, 21(4), pp. 523-8

Mullally, M et al. (2016). Anxiolytic activity and active principles of Piper amalago (Piperaceae) a medicinal plant used by the Q'eqchi' Maya to treat susto a culture-bound illness". J Ethnopharmacol (2016): 147-154. Doi:10.1016/j.jep.2016.03.013

Kikiuzaki, H et al. (1999). Antioxidative phenylpropanoids from berries of Pimenta dioica. Phytochemistry. Issue 52, pp.1307-1312

Marzouk, M. (2007). Anticancer and antioxidant tannins from Pimenta dioica leaves. Z Naturforsch. Jul-Aug, 62 (7-8), pp. 526-36

Jirovetz, L et al. (2007). Spice plants: Chemical composition and antioxidant properties of Pimenta Lindl essential oils, Part 1: Pimenta dioica (L) Merr. Leaf Oil from Jamaica. Nutrition. 31(2), pp. 55-63

Rao, P et al. (2012). An important spice, Pimenta dioica (Linn) Merill. International Current Pharmaceutical Journal. 1 (8), pp. 221-225

Zhang, L and Lokeshwar, B. (2012). Medicinal properties of the Jamaican pepper plant Pimenta dioica and Allspice. Curr Drug Targets. Dec, 13 (14), pp.1900-6

Klein, G et al.(2007). Antidiabetes and anti-obesity activity of Lagerstrormia speciosa. Evidence-Based Complement Alternat Medicine. December; 4 (4), pp. 401-407

Manish, A et al. (2010). In vitro antioxidant studies of Lagerstroemia speciosa leaves. Pharmacology Journal. June, vol 2 (10), pp. 357-361

Stohs, S et al. (2012). A review of the efficacy and safety of banaba (Lagerstroemia speciosa L) and corosolic acid. Phytother Res. March, 26 (3), pp. 317-324

Chan, E et al. (2014). Phytochemistry and Pharmacology of Lagerstroemia speciose: A natural remedy for Diabetes. Intl J Herbal Medicine. (2), pp. 100-105

Gracioso, J et al. (2002). Effects of tea from Turnera Ulmifolia L. on mouse gastric mucosa support the Turneraceae as a new source of anti-ulcerogenic drugs. Biol Pharm Bull. Apr; 25(4), pp. 487-491

Nascimneto, M et al. (2006). Turnera Ulmifolia (Turneraceae) preliminary study of its anti-oxidant activity. Bioresour Technol. Aug, 97(12), pp. 1387-91

Kumar, S and Sharma, A. (2007). Pharmacognostic investigations on Turnera ulmifolia. Nigerian Journal of Natural Products and Medicine. vol 11, pp. 5-9

Prabu, D et al. (2009). Effects of Turnera ulmifolia (Linn) Leaves on Blood Glucose Levels in Normal and Alloxan-induced Diabetic Rats. IJPT. July, vol 8(2), pp. 77-81

Sethi, P. (2011). Antibacterial activity of aqueous extract of the leaves of Turnera ulmifolia Linn (Turneraceae). ARPB. vol 1 (2), pp. 102-104

Brito, N et al. (2012). Antioxidant activity and protective effect of Turnera ulmifolia Linn var elegans against carbon tetrachloride-induced oxidative damage in rats. Food Chem Toxicol. Dec, 50 (12), pp. 4340-7

Raghu, C et al. (2004). In vitro cytotoxic activity of Lantana camara L. Indian J Pharmacol. 36, pp. 94-95

Nayak,S et al. (2008). Evaluation of wound healing activity of Lantana camara – A pre-clinical study. Phytother Res. vol 23 (2), pp. 241-45

Forestieri, A et al. (1996). Antiinflammatory, Analgesic and Antipyretic activity in rodents of plant extracts used in African medicine. Phytotherapy Research. vol 10, pp. 100-106

Sathish, R et al. (2011). Anti-ulcerogenic activity of Lantan camara leaves on gastric and duodenal ulcers in experimental rats. J Ethnopharmacol. Mar 8, 134(10), pp.195-197

Barreto, F et al. (2010). Antibacterial activity of Lantan camara Linn and Lantana montevidensis brig extracts from Carri-Ceara, Brazil. J Young Pharmacists. 2, pp. 42-4

Saxenam M et al. (2012). A brief review on therapeutical values of Lantana camara plant. Int J of Pharm and Life Sci (IJPLS). March, vol 3 (3), 1551-4

Kirimuhuzya, C et al.(2009). The anti-mycobacterial activity of Lantana camara, a plant traditionally used to treat symptoms of tuberculosis in South-Western Uganda. Afr Health Sci. March; 9 (1), pp. 40-45

Karita, S et al. (2012). A Review on Medicinal Properties of Lantana camara Linn. Research J. Pharm. and Tech. June 5 (6), pp. 711-715

Molina, M et al. (1999). Mimosa pudica may possess antidepressant actions in the rat. Phytomedicine. 6, pp. 319-23

Ngo Bum, E et al. (2004). Anticonvulsant activity of Mimosa pudica decoction. Fitoterapia. Jun, 75 (3-4), pp.309-14

Kokane, D et al. (2009). Evaluation of wound-healing activity of rootof Mimosa pudica. J Ethnopharmacol. July 15, 124 (2), pp. 311-314

Ahmad, H et al. (2012). Mimosa pudica L(Laajvanti): An Overview. Pharmacogn Rev. Jul-Dec, 6(12), pp.115-24

Gangully, M et al. (2007). Effect of Mimosa pudica root extract on vaginal estrous and serum hormones for screening of anti-fertility activity in albino mice. Contraception. Dec, 71 (6), pp. 482-5 www.hort.purdue.edu/newcrop/morton/soursop

Chang, F and Wu, Y. (2001). Novel cytotoxic annonaceous acetogenins from Annona muricata. J Nat Prod. July, 64 (7), 925-31

Adeyemi, D et al. (2008). Anti-hyperglycemic activities of Annona muricata (Linn). Afr J Tradit Complement Altern Med. Oct 25, 6 (1), pp. 62-69

Arthur, F et al. (2012). Evaluation of hepatoprotective effect of aqueous extract of Annona muricata (Linn) leaf against carbotetrachloride and acetaminophen-induced liver damage. 3, pp. 25-30

Moghadamtousi, S et al. (2015). Annona muricata (Annonaceae): A Review of its traditional uses, isolated Acetogenins and biological activities. Int J. Mol. Sci. July,16 (7). doi: 10.3390/ijms160715625

Brandao, M et al. (1997). Antimalarial activity of extracts and fractions from Bidens pilosa and other Bidens species (Asteraceae) correlated with the presence of acetylene and flavonoid compounds. J Ethnopharmacol. July, 57 (2), pp. 131-8

Hsu, Y et al. (2009). Anti-hyperglycemic effects and mechanism of Bidens pilosa water extract. J Ethnopharmacol. March 18, 122 (2), pp. 379-383

Nguelefack T et al. (2005). Relaxant effects of the neutral extract of the leaves of Bidens pilosa Linn on isolated rat vascular smooth muscle. Phytother Res. 19, pp. 207-210.

Nakama, S et al. (2012). Efficacy of Bidens pilosa extract against Herpes Simplex virus infection in vitro and in vivo. Evidence Based Complementary and Alternative Medicine.

doi: 10.1155/2012/413453

Sundararajan, P et al. (2006). Studies of anti-cancer and antipyretic activity of Bidens pilosa whole plant. Afr Health Sci. March, 6 (1), pp. 27-30

Imai,T et al. (2008). Heartwood extractives from the Amazonian trees Dipteryx odorata, Hymenaea coubaril and Astronium lecointei and their antioxidant activities. J Wood Sci. 54, pp. 470-475

Cecilio, A et al. (2012). Screening of Brazilian medicinal plants for antiviral activity against rotavirus. J. Ethnopharmacol. June 14, 141(3), pp. 975-81

Da Costa, M et al. (2014). Antifungal and cytotoxicity activities of the fresh xylem sap of Hymenaea coubaril L. and its major constituent fisetin. BMC Complementary and Alternative Medicine (2014); 14: 245. http://www.biomedcentral.com/ doi: 10.1186/1472-6882-14-245

Jaiswal, B. (2012). Solanum torvum: A Review of its Traditional Uses, Phytochemistry and Pharmacology. Int J Pharm Bio Sci. Oct, 3 (4), pp. 104-111

Nguelefack, T et al. (2008). Cardiovascular and anti-platelet aggregation activities of extracts from Solanum torvum (Solanaceae) fruits in rats. J Complement Integrat Med. vol 5, pp. 1-11

Peranginangin, J et al. (2013). Therapeutic potency of Solanum torvum Swartz on Benign Prostatic Hyperplasia (BPH): A Review. Int J Res Phytochem Pharmacol. 3(3), pp. 121-127

Simaratanamongkol, A et al. (2014). Angiotensin Converting Enzyme (ACE) inhibitory activity of Solanum torvum and isolation of a novel methyl salicylate glycoside. Journal of Functional Foods. doi:10.1016/j.jff.2014.08.014

Yousef, Z et al. (2013). Phytochemistry and Pharmacological Studies on Solanum torvum Swartz. J App Pharm Sci. April, 13(4), pp. 152-160

Andrade-Cetto, A and Cardenas-Vasquez, A. (2010). Gluconeogenesis inhibition and phytochemical composition of two Cecropia species. J Ethnopharmacol. vol 130 (1), pp. 93-97

Rojas, J et al. (2006). Screening for antimicrobial activity of ten medicinal plants used in Colombian folkloric medicine: A possible alternative treatment for non-nosocomial infections.

BMC Complementary and Alternative Medicine. 6:2. doi: 10.1186/1472-6882-6-2

Nicasio, P et al. (2005). Hypoglycemic effect and chlorogenic acid content in two Cecropia species. Phytother Res. 19 (8), pp. 661-64

Nayak, B. (2006). Cecropia peltata L. (Cecropiaceae) has wound-healing potential: A preclinical study in a Sprague Dawley rat model. Mar; 5(1), pp. 20-26

Robinson, R et al. (1990). Inactivation of Strongyloides stercoralis filariform larvae in vitro by six Jamaican plant extracts and three anthelmintics. W Indian Med Jour. Dec, 39 (4), pp. 213-217

Idu, M et al. (2007). Preliminary phytochemistry, antimicrobial properties and acute toxicity of Stachytarpheta jamaicensis (L) Vahl leaves. Trends Medical Research. 2, pp. 193-198

Alvarez, E et al. (2004). Inhibiting effect of leaf extracts of Stachytarpheta jamaicensis (Verbenaceae) on the respiratory burst of rat macrophages. Phytother Res. June, 18 (6), pp. 457-62

Okwu, D et al. (2010). Isolation and characterization of steroidal glycosides from the leaves of Stachytarpheta jamaicensis Linn. Vahl. Der Chemica Sinica. 1(2), pp. 6-14

Meena, R and Pitchai, R. (2011). Evaluation of antimicrobial activity and preliminary phytochemical studies on whole plant of Stachytarpheta jamaicensis (L) Vahl. Int Res J Pharm. 2 (3), pp. 234-239

Ikewuchu, J et al. (2009). Time course of the effect Stachytarpheta jamaicensis (L) Vahl has on plasma sodium and plasma potassium levels of normal rats. J Applied Sci Res. 5 (10), pp. 1741-1743

Liew, P and Yong, Y. (2016). Stachytarpheta jamaicensis (L) Vahl: From traditional usage to pharmacological evidence. Evidence Based Complementary and Alternative Medicine.

http://dx.doi.org/10.1155/2016/7842340

Kakade, A et al. (2008). A Comprehensive Review of Jatropha gossypifolia Linn. J Pharmacog Rev. vol 2 (4), pp. 2-6

Oduola, T et al. (2005). Mechanism of action of Jatropha gossypifolia stem latex as a haemostatic agent. Euro J Gen Med. 2(4), pp. 140-143

Panda, B et al. (2009). Antiinflammatory and analgesic activity of Jatropha gossypifolia in experimental animal models. Global J Pharmacol. 3(1), pp.1-5

Panda, B et al. (2009). Hepatoprotective activity of Jatropha gossypifolia against carbon tetrachloride-induced hepatic injury in rats. Asian J Pharm Clin Res. vol 2 (1), pp.50-54

Seth, R and Sarin, R. (2010). Analysis of the Phytochemical content and antimicrobial activity of Jatropha gossypifolia L. Arch Appl Sci Res. 2 (5), pp. 285-291

Devappa, R et al. (2011). Jatropha Diterpenes: A Review. J Am Oil Chem Soc. 88, pp. 301-322

Felix-Silva, J et al. (2014). Jatropha gossypifolia L. (Euphorbiaceae): A review of traditional uses, phytochemistry, pharmacology and toxicology of this medicinal plant. Evidence-Based Complementary and Alternative Medicine. http://dx.doi.org/10.1155/2014/369204

Sertie, J et al. (2000). Antiulcer activity of the crude extracts from the leaves of Casearia sylvestris. Pharm Bull. vol 38 (2), pp. 112-119

Oberlies, N et al. (2002). Novel bioactive clerodane diterpenoids from the leaves and twigs of Casearia sylvestris. J Nat Prod. Feb, 65 (2), pp.95-99

Borges, M et al. (2000). Effects of aqueous extract of Casearia sylvestris (Flacourtiaceae) on actions of snake and bee venoms and on activity of phospholipases A2. Comp Biol Physiol. Sept, vol 127 (1), pp. 21-30

Da Silva, S et al. (2008). Antimicrobial activity of ethanol extract from leaves of Casearia sylvestris. Pharm Biol. May, vol 46 (5), pp. 347-351

Schoenfelder, T et al. (2008). Antihyperlipidimic effect of Casearia sylvestris methanolic extract. Fitoterapia. Sept, vol 79 (6), pp. 465-7

Albano, M et al. (2013). Anti-inflammatory and antioxidant properties of hydroalcoholic crude extract from Casearia sylvestris Sw (Salicaceae). J Ethnopharmacol. March 29.

http://dx.doi.org/10.1016/j.jep.2013.03.049

Antinarelli, L et al. (2015). Antileishmanial activity of some Brazilian plants, with particular reference to Casearia sylvestris. An Acad Bras Cienc. 87(2), pp. 733-742

Websites

www.tropilab.com

www.plantamed.com.br

www.stuartxchange.com

www.hort.purdue.edu

www.hort.cornell.edu

www.ijptonline.com

Bibliography

Abbiw, D. (1990). Useful Plants of Ghana. Kew: Intermediate Technology Publishers & Royal Botanical Gardens

Ayensu, E. (1981). Medicinal Plants of the West Indies. Reference Publications Inc.

Brown, D. (1995). The RHS Encyclopedia of Herbs and Their Uses. BCA

Chevalier, A. (2000). Encyclopedia of Herbal Medicine. Dorling Kindersley

Duke, J. (1997). The Green Pharmacy. Rodale Press

Duke, J. (2009). Handbook of Medicinal Plants of Latin America. CRC Press

Fuglie L. (2001). The Moringa Tree: A local solution to malnutrition?' Dakar. CWS.

Harris, I. (2010). Healing Herbs of Jamaica. Ahha Press Inc.

Honeychurch, P. (1986). Caribbean wild plants & their uses. Macmillan Caribbean

Jaen, J. (1999). Canary Folk Medicine. Centro de la Cultura Popular Canaria

Marcu M. (2005). Miracle Tree. California. KOS Publications La Canada,

Robertson, D. (1982). Jamaican Herbs: Nutritional and Medicinal Values. Jamaican Herbs Ltd.

Rogans, E. (1997). Chinese Herbal Medicine. Element Books Ltd.

Solomon, N. (2002). Tahitian Noni Juice. Direct Source Publishing

Taylor, L. (2005). The Healing Power of Rainforest Herbs. Square One Publishers

Vogel, A. (1986). Nature – Your Guide to Healthy Living. Verlag A Vogel

White, L and Foster, S. (2000). The Herbal Drugstore. Rodale Books

Wren, R. (1998). Potters New Encyclopaedia of Botanical Drugs and Preparations. CW Daniel Company Ltd.

Printed by Amazon Italia Logistica S.r.l.
Torrazza Piemonte (TO), Italy

52525751R00071